PRAISE FOR *END TIMES HEALTH WAR*

In *End Times Health War*, Steve Wohlberg has taken a difficult and sometimes controversial subject and managed, by placing it in the setting of the war between good and evil, to create a near perfect blend of science, instruction, and spiritual insight that is practical and applicable to every one of us living on the planet today. His personal testimonies make for interesting, "bore-free" reading, his recommendations are medically defensible and wisely summarized, and his spiritual counsel absolutely essential if one hopes to realize the real and promised benefits assured. This is a masterpiece of health science that everyone interested in the very best possible health should read, digest, and, by the grace and power of God, apply.

Walter C. Thompson, MD
Author of *Health Smart: A Rational
No-Nonsense Practical Approach to Health*

I am a physician who has been in family practice for nearly 54 years, and I have been passionate about preventive medicine throughout my career. In August 2006, I chaired a committee in the city of Farmington, New Mexico that successfully banished smoking in the workplace. In more recent years, I have written and had published in my local newspaper, the Walla

Walla Union Bulletin, 82 articles on a variety of preventive medicine topics. A very high percentage of diseases are due to lifestyle choices and I feel certain that *End Times Health War* will make a great difference in the lives of those who read it.

Donald E. Casebolt, MD
Maryland

End Times Health War goes along with the belief that I've had for a long time that, as time goes by, the immune system of most people will be severely impaired. This explains the fact that in my practice I have been seeing a lot of young individuals (early 30s) develop diseases only known to older individuals (65-plus) 30 to 50 years ago. The most common cancer across the board in both males and females is lung cancer, and I see many individuals in their 30s dying of this dreaded disease. I believe one reason is due to the fact that their immune systems are so weakened because of the toxins mentioned in this book. *End Times Health War* couldn't have come in a more timely manner than now. Very insightful and informative. I highly recommend it to anyone interested in maximizing their health.

Joel Sabangan, MD, FCCP

Many Americans are waking up to the fact they now pay nearly all outpatient medical expenses. In short, they have nothing but catastrophic health care coverage. Thus, nearly all medical expenses for those under 65 will be out of pocket. It is timely that Steve Wohlberg's *End Times Health War* should be released now. As never before, it is time to get well and stay well at home. This book provides the information you need. I am well acquainted with the author, having stayed in his home and eaten at his table, and I assure you he has done also seen the incredible benefits of implementing exercise and the rest of the "eight natural doctors." We have witnessed firsthand an obese, wheelchair-bound lady lose over 100 pounds, get off about twenty medications, and achieve the ability to walk several miles. Many have lowered their cholesterol levels by 100 points. Reading this book could change your life!

LOREN MUNSON, MPT
JENNIFER MUNSON, MPT
Physical therapists and health educators

A jam-packed guide to organize and focus you on what is important and necessary to keep your mind and body in the best shape possible as we move through this uncertain and chaotic time just before Jesus Christ's return.

DONNA B. HELMICH, DDS

Steve Wohlberg is the kind of person who takes his health and life seriously. Because of that, when God brought new light into his life on His natural remedies, Steve took that information and applied it 100 percent. What a blessing for me to watch transformational healing take place in one who, even today, is unwilling to settle for anything less than God's best for his life—mentally, physically, and spiritually. Just as God offered this incredible privilege to Steve, He also waits to bestow that same healing balm to each of His precious children worldwide. After all, our health is a reflection on the God we serve. When we are healthy, others can see not only our Savior's loving character, but also His willingness and ability to graciously and abundantly care for His own. With our Lord's reputation on the line, our vibrant health is not just a nice idea—it's our commission to grasp His healing remedies extensive research into care of the human machine, making it easy for you to stay well at home and avoid a host of miracle cure mirages that entrap many Americans. While I appreciate that his book doesn't promote the sale of products or supplements, after reading his manuscript I still feel compelled to urge all Americans to take two supplements daily for the rest of their lives—vitamin D3 (I recommend 2000 to 4000 IU per day) and sublingual vitamin B12 (1000 to 2000 mcg per day), and don't rely on so-called "normal" reference ranges for these two. They can mislead to false security, with devastating injury to your health!

TIMOTHY JON ARNOTT, MD
Board-certified, Family Medicine
Founding Member, American College of Lifestyle Medicine

Too many people have grown comfortable letting their tongues dictate their food choices. Some are unaware of the toxins in our environment and food supply that contribute to illness. Some have traveled down the health road and failed. In *End Times Health War*, Steve Wohlberg gives new and fresh reasons and practical solutions for staying on track with good health practices. It's easier than most think. Concise, inspiring, readable, personal. A must-read for the seasoned health enthusiast or first timer.

DANIEL DREHER, ND
Director, Health Start

As physical therapists we can testify to the validity of the information presented in *End Times Health War*. In over 20 years of practice, we've witnessed the devastating results of preventable diseases caused by destructive lifestyles. We have and to be a living sacrifice. "I beseech you therefore, brethren, by the mercies of God, that you present your bodies a living sacrifice, holy, acceptable to God, which is your reasonable service" (Rom. 12:1). I wholeheartedly recommend *End Times Health War*.

LINDA CLARK
Director, Highway to Health

In *End Times Health War*, Steve Wohlberg reveals the solution that restored my health. I suffered from a toxin overload in 1993, which put me in bed for four months and on an 18-year search for recovery of health and energy. I found what I needed through the same wonderful and practical eight laws of health as well as the other nutrition information described in this book. My battle did not end the day I regained my health. I continue to breathe the air, eat the best organic food I can find, and drink pure water—but I still live in a toxic war zone called earth. To retain my health takes daily effort. *End Times Health War* is a powerful resource we all need, especially written for today's world.

SHERI YOHE
Author of *Add Life*, a gluten-free recipe book
and nutrition guide

END
TIMES
HEALTH
WAR

END TIMES HEALTH WAR

How to Outwit Deadly Diseases Through Super Nutrition and Following God's Eight Laws of Health

STEVE WOHLBERG

DESTINY IMAGE® PUBLISHERS, INC.
P.O. Box 310, Shippensburg, PA 17257-0310
"Promoting Inspired Lives."

This book and all other Destiny Image and Destiny Image Fiction books are available at Christian bookstores and distributors worldwide.

For more information on foreign distributors, call 717-532-3040.

Reach us on the Internet: www.destinyimage.com.

ISBN 13 TP: 978-0-7684-0453-1
ISBN 13 Ebook: 978-0-7684-0454-8

For Worldwide Distribution, Printed in the U.S.A.
2 3 4 5 6 7 8 / 18 17 16 15 14

DEDICATION

This book is dedicated to all who are sincerely seeking to improve their health, prevent disease, and stay alive in apocalyptic times. It is also dedicated to the One who created the human body to be the best doctor in town.

Contents

FOREWORD

Without a doubt, *End Times Health War* is a book for our time. Even casual observers realize that all is not well with Planet Earth, nor with the seven billion passengers on board. War rages today in every sense of the word, and Steve Wohlberg focuses our attention on some areas commonly overlooked. His book highlights the basics we must know to achieve optimal health, and also adds details frequently missed in other books of this genre.

Thirty-plus years of practicing family medicine and geriatrics and seeing thousands of patients has convinced me that traditional medicine by and large misses the mark in addressing the root causes of our patients' health problems. Based on my personal experience as a physician, I have become increasingly convinced that what my patients need is not another prescription, but critical information about how to overcome their diseases, plus encouragement to act upon that information. This book will provide you with that same information and give you the encouragement you need to dramatically change the course of your life for the better.

While *End Times Health War* clearly reveals how dangerous our world is, it won't leave you "shivering in the corner" afraid to move, but rather provides hope and practical solutions to today's health battles. It also carefully reveals where the real battles are being waged and how to be victorious in your own struggles against deadly foes, both seen and unseen.

It has been said that "necessity is the mother of invention" and that "where there's a will, there's a way." Steve Wohlberg's personal and family health challenges have been his "necessity" and "will" which have driven him to diligently search for both causes and treatments and have led to this book. Now you, the reader, have the opportunity to benefit from Steve's diligent quest for optimal health.

Enjoy the read. Practice the principles. Reap the benefits.

KEVIN BRYANT, MD, CMD
Family Practice/Geriatrics
Wichita, Kansas

INTRODUCTION

Not long ago I sat in a dentist's chair near my home in north Idaho. Flat on my back, I couldn't help overhearing this conversation. "There's a benefit dinner for Betty next week," my dentist reported to his assistant. "She has cancer. Her hair is falling out from the chemo which, while not a huge deal, hasn't made her too happy. Her brother has brain cancer too." *Oh my,* I thought quietly to myself, *is this Afghanistan? What a disease-filled minefield we live in. Will my own family survive the onslaught?*

That conversation between my dentist and his assistant reveals just the tip of the proverbial iceberg. I could relay many other stories, such as that of a four-year-old boy who was suddenly struck down with multiple malignant brain tumors. He's dead now. More than one of my friends has multiple sclerosis. Another died of liver disease. A teenage girl I know is battling Hodgkin's lymphoma. Just recently, I learned of another with bone cancer. A relative of mine died of a massive stroke at age thirty-two. I could go on and on. It's no secret that deadly diseases now stalk not only the elderly, but even small children. Unexpectedly, such illnesses often strike to kill. It's heartbreaking.

"People are dropping like flies," a close friend told me recently. He was right. Of course, I realize we all have to die sometime, but seriously, a four-year-old boy succumbing to brain tumors just doesn't seem normal. Nor a 32-year-old dropping dead from a massive stroke. These days, even kids are being diagnosed with blood, bone, and brain cancers.

What's going on?

In a nutshell, *we're at war.*

During World War I, total military and civilian deaths are generally estimated at around 16 million. During World War II, the count rose considerably. Over 60 million perished. During the Korean War, nearly 2 million died. In Vietnam, it was over 5 million. While estimates vary, deaths during the more recent Gulf, Iraq, Somalia, Afghanistan, and Syrian wars add more grisly statistics. But don't miss this sober fact: In a 2010 article entitled, "World Cancer Deaths to Double by 2030: UN," CBC News reported that the United Nations cancer agency now estimates that "cancer could kill more than 13.2 million people a year by 2030."[1] That's close to the toll of World War I and more than during the Korean and Vietnam wars combined—all in one year. "Cancer strikes one in two men and one in three women," reported Medscape Medical News.[2] When you add global fatalities related to obesity, hypertension, heart disease, stroke, diabetes, multiple sclerosis, osteoporosis, kidney and liver failures, Parkinson's, Alzheimer's, and dementia, the numbers are truly staggering.

Yes, bloody wars are horrifically tragic, but what most of us have to worry about isn't stray missiles, bullets, or roadside bombs, but dying early from deadly chronic diseases. It is this war that this book seeks to equip you to survive.

It's a war raging within our own cells.

It's an end-time war against our health.

The book of Daniel predicts that before the second coming of Jesus Christ humanity will enter a perilous period called "the time of the end" (Dan. 12:4). During that time, which I believe to be our own time, chronic lifestyle-related diseases will become rampant. Again, I realize we all have to die sometime, yet wise King Solomon once asked, "Why should you die before your time?" (Eccles. 7:17).

The goal of *End Times Health War* is to help you stay alive as long as possible. I repeat: cancer, heart disease, liver, kidney, and autoimmune diseases are killers. We're at war. As any intelligent soldier knows, facing a deadly enemy requires education, preparation, training, resolve, and commitment. We need these too. To avoid being lowered into a cold coffin "before our time," we must fight back by making extra efforts to strengthen our immune systems, which is the body's primary natural defense system against disease. And guess what? The good news is that we don't have to attend medical school to discover how to do it, because the key information is readily available to anyone committed enough to finding it.

Essentially, there are Eight Laws of Health that are as certain as the Pope is Catholic and the rabbi is Jewish that we may skillfully wield as weapons of defense to effectively combat invisible foes. They are:

1. Powerful nutrition

2. Regular exercise (even if it's just walking)

3. Drinking sufficient amounts of water

4. Health-enhancing sunlight

5. Saying "No!" to unhealthy practices

6. Breathing fresh air

7. Getting sufficient sleep, and finally

8. Keeping our consciences clean by living pure lives through faith in God.

If you look at the above list, honestly, which one of those eight principles do you think you can regularly violate without serious consequences? The truth is—not one of them. Beyond this, there are certain surefire ways to literally flood every one of our body's 50 to 100 trillion cells with super nutrition to give our immune systems an added boost. They aren't expensive either—eating more raw plant foods, juicing fresh fruits and vegetables (especially chlorophyll-rich greens), and even growing our own 100 percent organic live sprouts in our own homes for just pennies a day. This book will explain and document the incredible health benefits of each of these easy-to-follow protective measures and teach you exactly what to do.

So keep reading. Learn the facts. Fight for your health! If you listen and take heed to the end-time intelligence information in these pages, I promise you that at the very least you will significantly reduce your risk of dropping dead unexpectedly.

Next, you will feel better and more alive. Third, you'll save money too. Seriously, who doesn't want to live longer, become more productive, and enjoy life more fully with loved ones and friends? Don't you? I do. Most importantly, the life-or-death details in this book will enable you to provide better service to an infinite and all-wise God who not only carefully crafted the "fearfully and wonderfully made" (Ps. 139:14) house you live in (your body), but who daily sustains it "by the word of His power" (Heb. 1:3).

Don't ever forget this truth: the most important person to keep you healthy is not your doctor *but you*.

Consider this book as boot camp.

You can win this war—with God's help.

Chapter 1

WAR ZONE: MY OWN SON TARGETED

*War is much too serious a matter to be
entrusted to the military.*
—GEORGES CLEMENCEAU
(1841-1929), French statesman

I t all began on a beautiful summer day in July of 2007. My wife, Kristin, our three-year-old son, Seth, and I were peacefully driving down northern California's scenic Interstate Highway 101 among towering redwoods when calamity struck like lightning from a clear blue sky. "Something's wrong with Seth!" Kristin unexpectedly yelled after glancing backward at our child who had fallen asleep in his car seat just moments before. Immediately, I flashed a quick glance behind me (I was driving) and was shocked to see our little boy convulsing and jerking. Panic gripped me. Quickly, I pulled over, jumped into the back seat, and shook my son gently. "Seth? Are you having a bad dream? Wake up!"

He couldn't—he was having his first seizure.

Weeks later, he had a second seizure. Then a third. After numerous tests, more than one EEG, and an MRI, our son was finally diagnosed with a form of epilepsy and, based on the recommendation of three neurologists, was put on anti-seizure medication. "No known cause, no known cure," was the consistent conclusion we were given.

On the bright side, we were informed that Seth would probably outgrow this disorder by his teens, and we were firmly advised to "keep him on medication" until then, or until he went two years without a seizure and his brain produced a normal EEG. This was explained as standard protocol for his condition.

So, nervously—all the while fearing the possibility of harmful side effects—I began inserting into my trusting child's open mouth a high-powered brain drug twice a day for the next 16 months.

Things went reasonably well for about a year except for three unusual occurrences. First, Seth's breath smelled like rotten flesh every morning, which seemed highly abnormal in a child. Second, his sleeping patterns became increasingly erratic, causing him to jerk and bounce all over the bed each night. Third, my wife and I often watched in amazement and horror many nights as Seth would wake up and do weird things, such as contort his lips, mutter nonsense, cry uncontrollably, and wave both hands wildly near his ears as if he was being tormented by some unseen substance in his brain. Kristin and I eventually labeled these frightening occurrences "night events," and even recorded one on video. "It's nothing to worry about," our neurologist told us after watching our video clip. "These events have nothing to do with the medication."

In retrospect, we think he was wrong.

Then in October 2009, Seth had four more seizures—while on medication. Frantically, we drove him to Sacred Heart Children's Hospital in Spokane, Washington for another EEG. "His brain wave patterns are quite busy," reported the neurologist who read the report, "and he is not far away from having more serious seizures." Nevertheless, the official diagnosis remained the same: a form of epilepsy—no known cause, no known cure.

"You should increase his medication," our neurologist frankly informed us.

This troubled me greatly.

In the midst of my turmoil, floating up from somewhere deep within hazy memories was an ancient Bible passage that says, "the curse causeless shall not come" (Prov. 26:2 KJV). *There must be a cause to Seth's seizures,* I thought to myself, *and a solution.* "Dear God," I found myself praying from the depths of my aching soul, "please help me to discover *why* my little boy is having these awful seizures, and how to reverse this condition! In Jesus' name, amen." This was one of the most earnest prayers I have ever prayed in my entire life.

The full story is too lengthy to tell here; but in a nutshell, after that prayer I began doing my own homework. After typing "causes of seizures" on the Internet and after hours of research, I discovered that seizures can *sometimes* be caused by poisonous substances in the brain. On Wednesday night, October 14, 2009, Seth convulsed again, and the next day I faced an awful dilemma. *Should I fly to Bend, Oregon tomorrow for a weekend speaking appointment* (I am an ordained minister and travel frequently giving seminars on a variety of Bible topics) *or stay home with Kristin and Seth?* I was confused and tormented. I didn't want to leave my wife alone with a seizure-active child, but my seminar was pending. People were expecting me and depending on me.

Finally, on Thursday night I prayed. "Lord, if Seth has another seizure tonight, I'm not going." Thankfully, he didn't. So, I left, and I'm glad I did. For it was there, in Bend, Oregon, that I met a nutritionist who recommended a natural product called "PCA" specifically formulated by a brilliant chemist at Maxam Nutraceuticals to gently remove heavy metals from the body.

Hmm, I thought at first, *I don't know about this. Should I give this to Seth?* After purchasing a bottle, and then consulting with a sympathetic doctor friend who recognized each ingredient on the label, I decided to give it a try. I remember the exact date when we first sprayed PCA into Seth's mouth—October 29, 2009.

Amazingly, four nights later on November 1, something unusual happened. Seth lay sleeping right beside me as I was praying in our bedroom. Suddenly, a soft supernatural light seemed to fill my heart, and a vivid sense of peace flowed into me. That night, *for the first time in a long time,* Seth slept peacefully all night in one place without jerking about wildly during sleep.

Something is changing, I thought to myself. I was right.

As time went on, I realized more fully what was happening. This was war.

Chapter 2

WAR ZONE: NOW THE TARGET WAS ME

The greatest conflicts are not between two people,
but between one person and himself.
—GARTH BROOKS, American country musician

In the spring of 2011, while sitting in my office during a normal day at work, I suddenly began to feel dizzy. "I need to take a break," I said to a friend I had been visiting with. "I don't feel so well." He left, and then I took a walk. *What's going on?* I thought to myself. I was clueless.

After a while I felt better and dismissed the whole thing. Yet during my next Bible prophecy seminar held in Wichita, Kansas, the dizziness returned, along with some other frightening symptoms. My chest felt weird, and my strength lessened. During my second presentation (I was used to speaking four to five times during a weekend), I felt like I might pass out. I said nothing to my audience, took deep breaths in between sentences, and battled on. Somehow, I made it through the entire weekend.

The same thing happened in the fall during another speaking appointment in Florida, yet this time the symptoms were even worse. A tight chest. Weird feelings. Shots of pain. "Steve doesn't look good," said a medical professional in the audience to her husband as she observed me closely. Again, somehow I made it through the weekend. After my last talk, a group gathered around me, and someone took my blood pressure. It was quite high. How high, I don't remember.

Then came Thanksgiving Day 2011. My morning was normal, which I spent with my wife, Seth (now age 7), and our three-year-old daughter, Abby. Our plan was to eat Thanksgiving dinner with my wife's parents, who live nearby. Suddenly, as I was standing in our kitchen at about 9:00 a.m., I began to feel very strange, with pressure in my chest. It was worse than before. So much so that my first thought was that I might be having a heart attack. But after thinking for a few moments and evaluating everything, I made a split-second decision not to saying anything to Kristin or to call 911, but rather to go jogging. *This can't be a heart attack,* I comforted myself repeatedly. *I'm physically fit.* So, I quickly slipped on my running shoes and hit the road.

As I was hoping, the more I ran, the better I felt. *This wouldn't be happening if I was experiencing a heart attack,* I explained to myself. Of course, this was true. I jogged a few miles, felt much better, and returned home. Shortly thereafter, my family drove to Grandma's. A nurse was there too. I explained what happened, and she took my blood pressure. Again, it was quite high, but I don't remember the numbers.

Hmm, high blood pressure? I pondered. This was different. At age 52, I had never had hypertension before that I was aware of.

Before year's end, I filled one more speaking appointment in Bakersfield, California. There, I met a friendly nurse and explained my symptoms. Concerned, she kindly and promptly drove over to a nearby Walgreens and purchased a blood pressure monitor as a gift for me. Then she took my blood pressure. The numbers were somewhere around 160 to 170 systolic, over 90 or so diastolic. "You need to get those numbers down," she informed me, "closer to 120/80, which is normal." This sounded good to me. *I'll do my best,* I thought to myself.

At the end of December our family spent nearly a week with my mother and stepfather in sunny Palm Desert, California. I relaxed, sunbathed, ate well, and jogged regularly. No major symptoms. No chest pain. *Great!* I told myself, *perhaps I'm cured.*

Sorry, no such luck.

In early January, 2012, I was back at my office in north Idaho. At the end of a busy day, I felt a bit stressed. Returning home, out of curiosity I picked up my new blood pressure monitor, sat down, tried to calm down, and then took a reading. Pump, pump, pump. *Woosh.* At the end of the drill, I looked at the monitor. I remember those numbers exactly. 196 (systolic) over 116 (diastolic). *Oh my, oh my!* I thought in amazement, *this is serious.*

This time, I told my wife. "You should consider medication," she soberly replied with a look of deep concern. After researching the topic and discovering that prolonged hypertension would greatly increase my risk of developing heart or kidney disease, having a stroke, and a host of other problems,

I finally succumbed and entered the world of the medicated. This may sound strange to some of my readers, but up to that point, I had never been on any form of daily medication in my entire life. Overall, at age 52 I considered myself quite healthy. Now this. *What next?* I pondered ominously.

At the recommendation of a doctor friend of mine and out of pure desperation, in January 2012 I began taking Bystolic, a common blood pressure medication. At first, the dosage was small. It worked for a while, but then I was forced to increase the dose. Not only that, but I soon began to feel increased pressure in my hands and head. At night, my arms felt hot, and my hands felt bloated. Honestly, at times I felt like I was staring death in the face, and I was especially concerned about my ongoing ability to provide for my lovely wife and children.

In the weeks that followed, I tried to slow down at the office (FYI, I'm naturally a high-speed guy), improve my diet even more, and step up my exercise routine. But alas, my high blood pressure continued, which was a mystery to me, even while taking Bystolic. *Dear God, help me,* I prayed. Yet, as is often the case with our loving Lord, His answer didn't come right away. After a few months of taking Bystolic, I then added Lisinopril too. But alas again, I had to keep increasing the doses to keep my numbers down.

In June 2012, along with my associate Gilbert Navarro, I set out for another major speaking appointment at a large church event in Centralia, Missouri. By this time, I was getting desperate. After further research, I discovered that all high blood pressure medications, as effective as they may be, have side effects. Possibly dangerous ones. Here I was. Age 52. Supporting a family. On two medications. Needing to keep increasing the doses. Still feeling strange symptoms. Hot arms and bloated hands at night, with no relief in sight.

"Dear God!" I prayed quietly again at about 30,000 feet on an airplane, "You've just got to help me. I can't keep going on like this. When I get to Missouri, please lead me to someone who knows what to do! In the name of Jesus, amen."

Well, guess what? In Missouri, one morning when I wasn't speaking (this was a large event with many other speakers), Gilbert Navarro was manning our White Horse Media booth. A stranger approached him, introduced herself as Linda Clark, and said she was a proponent of natural healing. Soon I approached the booth, too, and spoke to Linda briefly. Then she walked away. "That woman believes in natural healing," Gilbert told me casually. "She left us some of her products." Fifteen minutes later a thought hit me. *Wait a minute. On the plane I prayed that God would guide me to someone in Missouri who could help me, and then this Linda Clark shows up. Maybe she is my answer to prayer.*

Immediately I went in search of this mystery woman. Entering the main auditorium, I scanned a crowd of perhaps three to four hundred. On the right side near the back, sitting with her husband I recognized the woman I had met briefly at our booth. Quietly slipping over to the row where she was sitting, I then asked her if we could visit privately outside for a bit, which she was happy to do. Back at our booth, I explained my high blood pressure situation in detail. After listening intently, I still remember her exact words. *"We can beat this,"* she said confidently. Unexpectedly, she then recommended something I hadn't thought of before—a raw juice fast.

"Hmm…okay," I replied.

At that point, I was willing to try anything that seemed reasonable.

So, upon returning home, on June 17, 2012 my juice fast began. It consisted mostly of raw carrots, celery, apples, lemons, beets, and kale (much of which came from my garden, which at that point was growing nicely), as well as plenty of water. I spoke by phone with Linda regularly, and she also sent me a steady supply of organic herbal products she said were designed to aid, nourish, detoxify, and invigorate my heart, veins, kidneys, liver, small intestine, colon, and central nervous system. To my supreme delight, after only three or four days into my fast, my blood pressure dropped to 110/63. *Wonderful,* I thought. Seeing real progress, I slowly weaned myself off Bystolic and Lisinopril. Then, on the morning of June 23, 2012, I took the plunge and became medication-free.

You'll never guess what happened next.

It was a beautiful spring day. Some friends were visiting with my family at our house in north Idaho. That afternoon, June 23, I felt the pressure rise. Yes, I really could feel it—in my veins and even in my temples. Slipping quietly away into our bedroom by myself, I grabbed my blood pressure monitor. Pump, pump, pump. *Woosh,* was the usual sound, as the air went out. Fearfully, I looked down—196, *which was awful,* over 76, *which was fabulous.*

Unbelievable, I thought to myself, *what a bizarre reading.* A high-risk upper number, and a perfectly healthy lower one.

I'm in a battle, I realized as never before. I was right.

Once again, the war was on.

Chapter 3

NO CAUSE, NO CURE?

All truths are easy to understand once they are discovered; the point is to discover them.
—GALILEO GALILEI, Italian physicist,
mathematician, astronomer

In November of 2009, shortly after Seth had his first good night's sleep in what seemed like ages (four nights after we began giving him the natural product PCA), I flew to Seattle, Washington for another weekend speaking appointment. On that Saturday night when my seminar was over, I struck up a conversation with a dentist friend of mine who had fallen into deep trouble during the early days of his practice. Mysteriously, he began to feel like he was losing his mind. "Then I found Dr. Jon Mundall," my dentist friend told me excitedly, "and he tested my body for heavy metals." The result was shocking. "I was loaded with mercury," he told me, "but fortunately, Dr. Mundall knew how to get the poison out." Then came a life-changing sentence from my friend's lips to my ears.

Looking at me eye to eye and speaking with the deepest earnestness, my dentist friend said with the utmost vigor, "Dr. Mundall gave me my life back!"

Wow, I thought. *I wonder if he can help Seth?* My friend thought so and promptly wrote down Dr. Mundall's phone number. The next day, I returned to north Idaho.

After discussing this with Kristin, we decided to contact Dr. Mundall right away. To my pleasant surprise, I learned that Dr. Mundall operated his Liberty Clinic in Spokane, Washington, not far from our home in Priest River, Idaho. I also learned that he was no novice. A graduate of Loma Linda University School of Medicine, Dr. Mundall's specialty was clinical toxicology. So I phoned his office, mentioned that I was referred by my dentist friend in Seattle, and we scheduled our first visit for December 4, 2009.

During that first appointment, not only did Dr. Mundall question the "no cause, no cure, keep Seth on medication" mantra we had so often heard, but he calmly recommended something no other neurologist had even hinted at, which was an analysis of Seth's vitamin, mineral, and heavy metal levels. We agreed, and then the doctor took samples of Seth's hair, blood, and urine, which were then sent to Doctor's Data Laboratory in Chicago.

A week or so later, the results came in. While shocking, they also confirmed my growing suspicions based on my research. Guess what? Seth's youthful body was *loaded with heavy metals like arsenic, uranium, cadmium, lead, cesium, antimony, barium, and a host of others poisons.* "These are neurotoxins," Dr. Mundall candidly informed us. "The combination is extremely bad, especially in children. They can definitely cause seizures."

As with my dentist friend, our new course was confirmed—*detoxification.*

In the weeks that followed, we continued using PCA, plus we added chelation therapy properly prescribed by Dr. Mundall. We also began supplementing Seth's diet with vitamins and minerals targeting his nerves and brain. On January 27, 2010, after following a carefully scheduled weaning process, we took the next big step. Contrary to the prevailing opinion of nearly every neurologist we had spoken to, *we took Seth entirely off his anti-seizure medication.*

The next three nights were absolutely awful. Each night, nearly one hour after falling asleep, Seth had another strange "night event" where he would wake up, scream uncontrollably, wave his hands near his ears, and roll around wildly. Temptation pressed hard upon us. *This is because you took Seth off his anti-seizure medicine.* Voices seemed to whisper relentlessly in our heads, *Put him back on the drug right away.* But, with Dr. Mundall's firm encouragement, we fought back, resisted those voices, and maintained a steady course.

On the fourth night, no night event. On the fifth and six nights, nothing again. But then about a week later, temptation struck hard again. Seth had two more seizures back to back. "Hold the line," Dr. Mundall persisted. "These are side effects of *getting off the medicine,* not a reason to go back." It was exceedingly difficult, but we stuck it out.

Our persistence was rewarded.

In the weeks that followed, those bizarre "night events" ceased entirely and Seth's sleeping patterns steadily improved. Then came the kicker. On February 2, 2010, we returned to Sacred Heart Children's Hospital in Spokane, Washington for a follow-up EEG after the one he had approximately four months earlier in October. Three weeks later a neurologist (not Dr. Mundall) reported the results to our family physician: Seth's brain activity had significantly changed for the better, so much so that the former diagnosis was reversed. He *no longer* had any form of epilepsy. Praise God!

As I write this (it's now June 2014), Seth remains off all medication, hardly ever has "night events," and sleeps peacefully almost every night. I would be lying if I said there haven't been any bumps along the road, but based on the big picture Kristin and I know we're on the right track, and I can't tell you what a relief this has been to our family.

Now let me clarify something. I'm certainly not against doctors (Dr. Mundall is a doctor), nor am I angry with the other neurologists I had spoken to. Nevertheless, this trying experience taught my family that even sincere medical professionals can sometimes miss the boat by: 1) not searching for the underlying cause of a disease, and 2) being clueless about how to correct it. In Seth's case, a powerful brain drug was consistently recommended, but there was a better, more natural way.

Prior to Seth's February EEG, I told my wife, "Honey, if Seth's next EEG shows major improvement from the one in October (during the interim we were using PCA and focusing on detox with Dr. Mundall), I'm going public with our story." Thankfully, it did. So in April of 2010, I finally wrote down the details of our family's journey in an article entitled "No Cause, No Cure?" which I then not only posted on our White Horse Media website, but also emailed to my entire e-news list of nearly 7,000 recipients. The response was phenomenal.

Hundreds emailed me back requesting more information, and many of these shared their own stories of mysterious struggles, illnesses, and seizures.

One particular story stands out in my mind. It came from a woman living in Europe. She had cancer, and after turning toward natural healing, she went through a major detoxification protocol to strengthen her body to fight back. "One night, at about 4:00 a.m.," she informed me in an email, "my husband told me that this awful stench poured out of my body as I lay sleeping right next to him. He said it smelled like heavy metals." I distinctly remember this email because the exact same thing happened to Seth. During a period of heavy detox, one night at about 4:00 a.m. as he lay sleeping beside me in the same bed, I smelled an awful odor too. Following the scent, I discovered it was coming from Seth. It seems that the body picks certain times to dump chemicals, and perhaps 4:00 a.m. is one of them.

"How did your little boy get so much lead, arsenic, cadmium, and uranium in his body?" was the most common question I was asked by those who read our story.

I'll answer that question shortly.

But first, I'll increase the mystery by saying that in June of 2010 our entire family (me, Kristin, Seth, and our two-and-a-half-year-old daughter, Abby) went back to Dr. Mundall's Liberty Clinic to be tested for heavy metals. As a 50-plus man who grew up in Los Angeles, California, I was quite keen to see what chemicals might be lurking inside my brain too. *Snip, snip,* went Dr. Jon Mundall with his scissors. After placing hair strands from each of our heads into plastic bags, he sent them to Doctor's Data.

Four weeks later, my results came in. "Elevated levels of lead, cadmium, arsenic, and uranium"—the same substances we found were in Seth. What about little Abby? Are you ready for this? *Same thing.* She was loaded. In fact, Abby turned out to be the most toxic member of our family! Not only that, but after we started chelation therapy for her too, one day her diaper had the most awful odor, unlike any other. Kristin smelled it too. *It smelled like heavy metals.* How is this possible? How can apparently healthy children become so grossly contaminated?

You're about to find out.

Chapter 4

END TIMES REPORT: PLANET EARTH IS TOXIC

There's so much pollution in the air now that if it weren't for our lungs there'd be no place to put it all. —ROBERT ORBEN, AMERICAN COMEDIAN

Beginning in October of 2009 when Seth had a series of awful seizures and a highly erratic EEG, I have done ongoing research about toxic chemicals in the environment and their possible connection to increasingly rampant woes like autism, seizures, Alzheimer's, Parkinson's, multiple sclerosis, and even cancer. Can you blame me? I just had to help my son. In my earnest quest for knowledge, I read each of these eye-opening books (plus many others):

- *Detoxify or Die*, by Dr. Sherry Rogers, MD

- *Invisible Killers: The Truth about Environmental Genocide*, by Rik Deitsch and Dr. Stewart Lonkey, MD

- *Excitotoxins: The Taste That Kills*, by Dr. Russell L. Blaylock, MD

- *The Hundred-Year Lie: How to Protect Yourself from the Chemicals That Are Destroying Your Health*, by Randall Fitzgerald

Personally, I think it would be wise for you to consider reading some of these books. Read the customer reviews on amazon.com. For the record, I'm not saying I agree with every sentence; but overall, the information is solid. "Where did your boy get all those poisons?" Now I know. As you are about to discover too, they come from breathing, eating, living in modern homes, and playing with toys most kids play with. In other words, from twenty-first-century polluted air, water, soil, and supermarkets. Even from the personal care products we use every day like shampoo, conditioner, deodorant, soap, and toothpaste. "If more than used for brushing is accidentally swallowed," says the fine print on most name-brand tooth-pastes, "get medical help or contact a Poison Control Center right away."

Poison Control Center because of swallowing toothpaste? I don't know about you, but this doesn't sound good to me.

It's common knowledge that fish—both salt-water and fresh—are often loaded with mercury. Unfortunately, their slimy bodies aren't the only ones contaminated. Ours have been invaded, too. The fact is, whether we realize it or not, you and I now have the unfortunate privilege of being official members of the most toxic generation in the history of the world. We're all victims. There's no escaping it. Don't forget, we're in "the time of the end" (Dan. 12:4), and this is war. Just like the famous Greek legend of the Trojan horse, the enemy often sneaks in without our knowing it.

If you're not convinced, first consider this. In 1997, a series of articles published in *The Seattle Times* called "Fear in the Fields: How Hazardous Waste Becomes Fertilizer" gave this shocking report:

> A *Seattle Times* investigation found that, across the nation, industrial wastes laden with heavy metals and other dangerous materials are being used as fertilizer and spread over farmland. The process, which is legal, saves dirty industries the high costs of disposing of hazardous wastes.[3]

In his eye-opening book, *Fateful Harvest*, Pulitzer Prize finalist Duff Wilson first investigates and then documents this largely secretive and dangerous practice. As unbelievable as it sounds—it's happening. Across North America, hundreds of large industrial and chemical companies, such as Big Steel, Big Aluminum, and Big Coal, are now saving Big Bucks by disposing billions of tons of poisonous toxic wastes—not by sending them to landfills, which they should be doing (but which is expensive), but by cost effectively reclassifying them as "products" that aren't regulated by the EPA, and then by selling them as "bulk soil amendments" to unsuspecting fertilizer companies.

These harmful toxins then enter farming soils, commercially-grown plants, and the food chain.

Then they enter *you and me*.

It's a toxic trade, and most farmers don't even know what's going on under their noses. Yet it's a fact. Poisonous wastes *are* silently seeping from big industry onto railcars, into fertilizer companies, and then onto farmland, gardens, and crops like potatoes, corn, wheat, and soybeans. Unknowingly, when we innocently purchase produce from our local supermarket, these deadly chemicals (which don't appear on *any* labels) often slip silently into *our bodies and those of our kids.*

Outrageous, isn't it?

For proof, read Wilson's book.

On July 3, 2010, I spoke about what I have come to call "toxic terrorism" in Chewelah, Washington, not far from our home in northern Idaho. "Here's my story," said a woman after hearing my presentation, "I'm a farmer, and some time ago I visited another farmer in Rosalia, Washington, who farms thousands of acres of wheat. I noticed that there were no gophers on his land. 'What's your secret?' I asked my friend. His response amazed me. 'My soil contains so many chemicals that no gopher lives here.' Then he added, 'There's not even a worm on my land.' That's when the lights went on in my head about what's happening."

Dumfounded, I then asked this lady, "What happens to all that wheat? Is it harvested to feed animals?"

"No," she quickly retorted, "it goes into the whole wheat bread we purchase in markets." How frightening! I can't help but wonder whether this might contribute to increasingly common "wheat intolerances."

My wife now makes our own bread from organic wheat.

If you're still skeptical and really want to have your eyes opened to the vast extent of toxicity invading every one of us, visit YouTube.com and search for a series of presentations called "Ten Americans," produced by the Environmental

Working Group. Ken Cook, the president, is the featured speaker. I strongly recommend that you watch those videos. At the beginning of Mr. Cook's presentation, he pleasantly explains how his organization chose ten random Americans, took samples of their blood, and then subjected those samples to rigorous testing. The result? In each and every person they found:

- 212 industrial chemicals and pesticides

- 47 well-known consumer product ingredients

- 134 chemicals that are known carcinogens

Mr. Cook's audience could scarcely believe their ears. Mr. Cook then inquired, "Where did these ten random Americans get all these poisonous chemicals?" Then he threw a curve ball. After describing how many dangerous chemicals there are in everyday air (especially in cities), he stumped his hearers by saying, "Not from the air." *What?* Next he mentioned the pollutants saturating tap water. "Not from the water," he continued. *What?* Once more. Next he described the myriads of poisons found in grapes, strawberries, potatoes, apples, etc. due to chemical agricultural farming practices. "But they didn't get them from their food," Mr. Cook explained.

How can this be?

His audience sat spellbound.

Pushing the remote advancer for his PowerPoint presentation, Mr. Cook then showed a photograph of an ultrasound peering inside a woman's body. "That's my son before his birth," Mr. Cook declared, becoming visibly choked up. "He was one of those ten Americans." He then explained that the ten Americans were all fetuses whose umbilical cord blood had been closely analyzed by specialists *before they were born.*

Get it?

These poisons are in all of us.

Like I said, we have the unfortunate privilege of being official members of the most toxic generation in the history of the world. Can these chemicals destroy our health? *Click.* Mr. Cook pushed his button, and there appeared on the screen the innocent face of a young child who looked to me like a four-year-old. Below that face appeared this startling statistic: "57 percent increase in childhood brain cancer."

It's enough to make one weep.

In July 2010, Medline Plus, a service of the U.S. National Library of Medicine and the National Institutes of Health, listed cancer as the third-leading cause of death among children, ages one to four, and as the second-leading cause of death among children ages five to fourteen.[4] The U.S. Center for Disease Control's (CDC) "Fourth National Report on Human Exposure to Environmental Chemicals" reiterates Ken Cook's research by stating that the CDC report "presents exposure data for 212 environmental chemicals…in blood and urine. The Fourth Report includes results for 75 chemicals measured for the first time in the U.S. population."[5]

Like I said, we're all toxic.

If these chemicals were fluorescent, we'd glow in the dark.

As I mentioned in my Introduction, I know of a four-year-old boy who ended up in a coffin. I learned of this tragedy during one of my seminars discussing Bible prophecy and "the last days" (see 2 Tim. 3:1). A few months earlier, from what I was told, this little guy appeared normal and healthy.

Suddenly, he started having seizures. When doctors took a closer look, they were horrified to discover that the boy's brain was riddled with malignant tumors. Soon he was dead.

While the exact details of what caused those tumors remains a mystery, I now know that environmental toxins *can* cause tumors. Make no mistake about it—toxic terrorism is real, serious, and deadly. Check out these facts straight from the EPA:

1. Mercury impairs neurological development (especially in children) and damages the brain.[6]

2. Lead affects practically all systems of the body, especially the central nervous system, kidney, and blood cells. It can cause convulsions, coma, and death.[7]

3. Arsenic has been linked to cancer of the lungs, bladder, skin, kidneys, liver, and prostate.[8]

4. Uranium damages the kidneys and increases risk of bone, lung, and liver cancers, plus blood diseases.[9]

5. Cadmium affects the heart and blood vessels, GI tract, nervous, urinary, reproductive, and respiratory systems, and causes cancer.[10]

Are you beginning to realize that this is war?

If not, wake up! Sleeping soldiers are easy targets.

Unfortunately, the above tiny list is just the beginning. According to a series of articles published by *Scientific American* called "Chemical Marketplace," there are more than

80,000 chemicals produced and used in the US alone.[11] How many are carcinogenic? Only God knows.

I confess, I'm a minister, not a doctor; but after discovering such sober facts about the extent of the chemical soup that surrounds us and its potential effects upon our health, I began to search God's Word to see if it made any predictions about end-time toxicity. Allow me to share some pertinent Bible verses. The prophet Isaiah predicted that eventually:

> *The earth mourns and fades away, the world languishes and fades away; the haughty people of the earth languish* (Isaiah 24:4).

This passage predicts that "the earth" itself would mourn, fade away, and languish. To me, this suggests an environmental crisis of the worst sort, which I think applies especially to "the time of the end" (Dan. 12:4)—the time we live in now. Here's another one. The Lord told Isaiah:

> *The earth will grow old like a garment, and those who dwell in it will die in like manner* (Isaiah 51:6).

Similar to Isaiah 24:4, this passage describes "the earth" growing "old," but then it advances to the prediction that "those who dwell in it will die in like manner." In other words, as "the earth" itself slowly disintegrates as a consequence of sin, its inhabitants will suffer and die as a direct result of this aging process. Again, this fits perfectly with global environmental pollution, the poisoning of our oceans through catastrophes like the Fukushima nuclear disaster pumping radioactive contaminants into the Pacific Ocean, massive oil and chemical spills, deforestation, wide-scale soil depletion of organic matter and trace minerals due to commercial agricultural practices, pesticide overuse, the deadly poisoning of air, especially in large cities, and the so-called "acid rain" that results—all of which have harmful effects upon human health.

Open your eyes. Untold numbers are perishing due to earth's toxic woes. And it's not just humans. Have you heard about mass animal die-offs? In the spring of 2012, I was featured in a National Geographic International documentary entitled *Animal Armageddon,* which documents the recent and unusual uptick of mass deaths of birds, fish, bats, dolphins, and whales worldwide. Especially bees. Have you heard of colony collapse disorder? The cover of the August 19, 2013 issue of *Time* pictured a lone honeybee just below the sober headline, "A World without Bees: The Price We'll Pay If We Don't Figure Out What's Killing the Honeybee." The feature story reported:

> You can thank the Apis Mellifera, better known as the Western honeybee, for 1 in every 3 mouthfuls of food you'll eat today. ...Honeybees "are the glue that hold our agricultural system together," wrote journalist Hannah Nordhaus in her 2011 book, The Beekeeper's Lament. ...Honeybees are still dying on a scale rarely seen before, and the reasons remain mysterious. One-third of U.S. honeybee colonies died or disappeared during the past winter, a 42% increase over the year before and well above the 10% to 15% losses beekeepers used to experience in normal winters.[12]

What's causing this catastrophe? According to current research, probably pesticides, which "are used on more than 140 different crops as well as in home gardens." In a sidebar, these words appeared in bold letters:

> The take-home message is that we are very close to the edge. It's a roll of the dice now. —Jeff Pettis, USDA[13]

Ominously, the *Time* article also noted:

> The loss of honeybees would leave the planet poorer and hungrier, but what's really scary is the fear that bees may be a sign of what's to come, a symbol that something is deeply wrong with the world around us. "If we don't make some changes soon, we're going to see disaster," says Tom Theobald, a beekeeper in Colorado. "The bees are just the beginning."[14]

"Just the beginning"? Sounds apocalyptic to me. The last book of the Bible makes a startling prediction. The context is clearly "the end of days." Notice carefully:

> *The nations were angry, and Your wrath has come, and the time of the dead, that they should be judged, and that You should reward Your servants the prophets and the saints, and those who fear Your name, small and great, and should destroy those who destroy the earth* (Revelation 11:18).

This end-time prophecy informs us that at the sunset of human history, God Almighty will finally intervene—and His act will come at a time when misguided mankind is literally destroying His green earth. To be perfectly clear, I'm no rabid environmentalist (although I deeply appreciate the planet our Creator made for us); but to me, these Bible predictions pinpoint *our generation*. Now here's the kicker. Revelation also warns:

> *Woe to the inhabitants of the earth and the sea! For the devil has come down to you, having great wrath, because he knows that he has a short time* (Revelation 12:12).

It's obvious that Big Chemicals, Big Agriculture, Big Pharmaceuticals, Big Politics, and even Big Government often yield to the temptation to crave financial profit above an unselfish interest in human health. But is it possible that there is also a highly intelligent and malicious force operating *invisibly* behind the scenes bent on corrupting complex human DNA strands within our cells, undermining human immune systems, polluting human bloodstreams, manipulating and controlling human minds, and destroying human souls? The Bible says there is. It is "the Devil and Satan, who deceives the whole world" (Rev. 12:9). *He* is the ultimate inspiration behind human brutality, the gradual destruction of Planet Earth, and toxic terrorism.

Take note. Revelation 12 is a war chapter. Beginning with a war in heaven (see verse 7), it chronicles the progress of the Great Controversy between God and His former top angelic chief officer throughout history, culminating at the end. "Woe to the inhabitants of the earth and the sea," warns Bible prophecy. Yes, Lucifer exists, and he is not only warring against our souls (trying to keep us from God) but against our brains, bones, and bodies too. Indeed, he is the primary foe behind the global end-times war against our health.

Let me clarify. I don't believe that Satan himself is directly injecting millions of tons of formaldehyde, sulfur dioxide, dioxins, sodium laurel sulfate, PCBs, DDT, Agent Orange, radiation, and heavy metals like mercury, arsenic, lead, and uranium into our environment, but I do believe he is working *invisibly* behind the scenes through many chemical companies and corporate profiteering to poison humanity. Just like he first spoke through a serpent in Eden, so he works today through agents (and agencies—even government ones) "to steal, and to kill, and to *destroy*" (John 10:10).

"He was a murderer from the beginning," warned Jesus Christ (John 8:44).

He is a murderer today.

Thankfully, God still rules from in the heavens, and He is much stronger than the prince of poisons. The more I research this topic, the more impressed I am at how the Great Physician is working to help humanity survive the deadly forces arrayed against us. Even though physical healing rarely happens instantly, during these past few years my son's condition has steadily improved, and his smiling face brings joy to my heart every day. "I had lead in my head!" Seth blurted out once with a boyish twinkle. With God's help, combined with healthy choices, I'm determined that my son will not become another cancer statistic. I hope not. I pray not.

Or my wife. Or Abby. Or me.

Let me clarify something else. When I sometimes use the phrase *toxic terrorism* in my weekend seminars, I use the word *terrorism* because many of the invading chemicals we're exposed to daily are literally *at war with normal DNA functions, our immune systems, vital organs, brains, and minds—and consequently with our relationship with God.*

It was Halloween evening, 1938. Orson Welles began narrating H.G. Wells' book, *The War of the Worlds,* to his unsuspecting radio audience. "Hostile invaders have come from Mars," the announcer stated, "and have landed in New Jersey. The eerie creatures are marching forward rapidly, killing as they go. Great destruction is taking place!" Fear gripped listeners who thought it was real. "Fake Radio War Strikes Terror across America," ran newspaper headlines the next day.

Obviously, that narrated book in 1938 was just a story, but today's silent invasion of deadly pollutants into our mouths, skin, lungs, livers, kidneys, bones, blood, and brains isn't. Again, the threat is real, as are the tumors, cancers, and frightening diseases often related to them. Is there anything we can do to protect ourselves and our loved ones against this diabolic onslaught? Thankfully, yes, there is. Although we can't stop the invasion entirely, there are nevertheless some solid principles, practices, foods, and liquids that will enable our bodies to effectively fight these infernal foes. We *can* escape an early encounter with the Grim Reaper. We *can* avoid dying before our time (see Eccles. 7:17).

Heaven has provided powerful weapons of defense.

It's time to begin discovering those weapons that can literally save our lives and the lives of those we love.

Chapter 5

PUT ON THE WHOLE
ARMOR OF GOD

*The truth that makes men free is for the most
part the truth that men prefer not to hear.*
—HERBERT AGAR (1897-1980),
American author, journalist

"Put on the whole armor of God," urged Paul in the New
Testament, "that you may be able to stand against the
wiles of the devil" (Eph. 6:11). Then he wrote a list of heavenly weaponry. The first is, "Stand therefore, having girded
your waist with *truth*" (Eph. 6:14). Of course, "truth" applies
to many areas, such as true doctrines; the truth about divine
creation (see Gen. 1:1); the truth about the existence, rebel-
lion, and fall of Lucifer (see Rev. 12:9); the truth about human
sin and the fall of man (see Gen. 3; Rom. 3:23); and the
truth about our desperate need for a Savior to restore our lost
estate (see Matt. 1:21). Yet the word *truth* also applies to certain fixed, immovable, and immutable laws of health which,

once discovered and followed, will greatly aid us soldiers as we battle fierce unseen foes seeking to destroy our bodies, our happiness, and our lives. Before listing those laws, here are some health-related truths that are extremely helpful for us to understand.

TRUTH: WE HAVE BEEN CREATED BY GOD

"In the beginning God created the heavens and the earth" (Gen. 1:1), declares the very first sentence of the world's all-time number-one bestselling book. "So God created man in His own image; in the image of God He created him; male and female He created them" (Gen. 1:27). According to the Holy Scriptures, humanity didn't burst on the scene due to some ancient, cosmic Big Bang or evolve over trillions of years from accidental, haphazard, mindless goop; we sprang into existence from the holy hand of a Master Designer, God Himself. "I am fearfully and wonderfully made" (Ps. 139:14), penned David.

In their fascinating book, *Darwin's Demise: Why Evolution Can't Take the Heat*, Dr. Joe White and Dr. Nicholas Comninellis unveil these incredible facts about the physical body we take so much for granted:

- The human eye can handle 1.5 million simultaneous messages.

- A single inner ear contains as many circuits as the telephone system of a large city.

- The DNA of even a single microscopic human cell is composed of 3 billion units and contains all the information necessary to construct an entire adult human.

- The brain has 10 billion circuits and a memory of 1 sextillion bits. With its 12 billion brain cells and 120 connections, it's the most complex arrangement in the universe.[15]

Honestly, can random "chance" account for such exquisite organization? I don't think so. To me, the sheer wonder of our bodies, brains, cells, and systems totally negates the notion of evolution from monkeys. *Incomprehensible complexity* is the phrase used by some scientists to describe the incredible orchestration of life. Human beings—including you and me—are not the result of Darwinian "survival of the fittest." Instead, the sublime *truth* recorded in the Scriptures is:

> *The hearing ear and the seeing eye, the Lord has made them both* (Proverbs 20:12).

TRUTH: OUR CREATOR WANTS US TO BE HEALTHY, NOT SICK

The apostle John wrote to his Christian converts, "I pray that you may prosper in all things and *be in health*, just as your soul prospers" (3 John 2). There it is. Writing by divine inspiration, John declared that he wants us to "be in health." But the ultimate proof that possessing a healthy body is God's will for every human being can easily be detected by examining the earthly life of Jesus Christ. Notice carefully:

And Jesus went about all Galilee, teaching in their synagogues, preaching the gospel of the kingdom, and healing all kinds of sickness and all kinds of diseases among the people. Then His fame went throughout all Syria; and they brought to Him all sick people who were afflicted with various diseases and torments, and those who were demon-possessed, epileptics, and paralytics; and He healed them (Matthew 4:23-24).

Thus Jesus Christ was not only a Teacher, Preacher, and Savior, but a Heavenly Healer too. During His life on earth, He hated to watch humans suffer, so with a divine/human touch He banished every form of disease. Even devils fled from His power. Now that He has died for our sins (see 1 Cor. 15:3), been raised from the dead (see Matt. 28:1-7), and ascended bodily to heaven (see Acts 1:9-11), He has lost none of His compassionate nature. True, He doesn't always heal human ills today in openly miraculous ways, but we can be sure that His loving heart remains unchanged. "Jesus Christ is the same yesterday, today, and forever" (Hebrews 13:8), says the Holy Book.

My point is this: *God wants us to be healthy,* that's for sure.

TRUTH: FANTASTIC HEALTH FLOWS FROM A COMBINATION OF HEALTHY CHOICES

Here's a wise saying worth remembering: "Good health is an *orchestra,* not an instrument." In other words, real health won't happen from one pill, one potion, one product, one formula, or even from one food. Sorry. It just doesn't happen that way. Vibrant health is the reward of an orchestra of healthy decisions. Let me explain.

Think of a living plant growing in a pot on your sundeck. You may pour fertilizer on its base, but if you then place the pot in a dark closet the plant will die. If you place it back on the sundeck but never water it, it will still wither away. Even if it gets plenty of water and sunlight but if you pluck it from its soil, it's doomed. Make sense? Plants are like people. To be healthy, we need a *combination* of pure water, whole food nutrition, proper amounts of sunlight, fresh air, regular exercise, moderation in work, times of relaxation, and a soothing night's sleep (we will explore each of these health-enhancers more fully soon). If we do most of these but then relentlessly push ourselves to remain awake past midnight regularly, at some point we'll crack.

Never forget this truth: *real health is the rich reward of a combination of healthy choices.* So don't be fooled by slick ads promoting this-will-cure-everything gadgets, formulas, or pills.

Again, one product alone won't cut it.

Truth: To Enjoy Good Health, We Must Obey Nature's Laws

Think of gravity. What goes up comes down, not just in America, but in China too. Back to plants. Plants need soil, water, fresh air, and sunshine whether they grow in Australia or South Africa. Yes, variety exists, but all within the context of fixed universal laws. It's the same with our health. There are health laws too—laws that have been firmly established by our Creator Himself. Consider exercise. Taking a pleasant walk will benefit anyone, whether one's skin is black, white, brown, red, or yellow. Or sleep. We all need it, whether Russian or British.

Vitamin C not only helped European sailors avoid scurvy, but it's necessary for athletes, mechanics, computer programmers, CEOs, and movie stars. Cigar smoking increases the risk of lung cancer, whether a person lights up in Paris, Peru, or Los Angeles.

Whether we like it or not, there's no escaping it.

Fixed health laws exist.

If we obey natural laws, we will reap improved health. If we don't, we'll pay a painful price. "Whatever a man sows, that he will also reap" (Gal. 6:7). Therefore, to discover and obey these laws should be one of our top priorities. Remember that Bible verse that floated into my mind when I prayed for Seth? "The curse causeless shall not come" (Prov. 26:2 KJV). Whether we realize it or not, every illness has *a cause* somewhere, and that cause *always* has something to do with breaking natural laws. If we are sick, our challenge is to seek to identify that cause—which isn't always easy—and to correct it, if possible, so we can return to harmony with the laws of life.

Why are so many of us sick today? Obviously, disease is often complicated, and sickness usually involves a subtle interplay between genetics, environment, and choices. That said, here are some "lifestyle-related" clues that help explain global woes: cigarette puffing, alcohol guzzling, caffeine cravings, drug use and abuse (illegal and prescription), soda pop, junk food, lazy living, loud music, overeating, overwork, stressful days, wild nights, tired bodies, and little sleep. As we consider how common these are, is it any wonder many of us are falling apart at the seams? Again, "the curse causeless shall not come" (Prov. 26:2 KJV). There *are* causes to human illness. In the mad rush to fatten our wallets and find fast thrills, all too many of us—without realizing it—violate nature's laws, which are really God's laws. "You shall not murder" (Exod. 20:13), thundered an Almighty Lawgiver from His mountain pulpit (Mount Sinai), which also applies to self-murder by unhealthy habits. To be blunt, when we violate nature's health laws, we sin against God and ourselves.

Sadly, humanity is now doing this regularly, 24/7.

"All have sinned" (Rom. 3:23), says the Lord.

Truth: Our Bodies Have Natural Detoxification Systems

Once, I posted a note on my Facebook page about the benefits of detoxification and was amazed to read a rather critical response from a friend, who happens to be a nurse. Essentially, she stated that the whole "detox" notion is a myth. Now, I realize that there are plenty of detox-quick scams skillfully marketed merely to make a buck, but really. Detox itself—a scam?

Consider this: The deeper we delve into the intricacies of human anatomy, the more we discover the marvelous truth that our bodies have been exquisitely created with natural detoxification systems highly capable of eliminating poisons and fighting disease. Each of us has an incredibly complex immune system able to identify, tag, form antibodies against, and then finally zap hostile invaders; a liver (which is a detox powerhouse); two kidneys (which constantly filter poisons from our bloodstreams); a large bowel (you know what that's for);

and permeable skin that is constantly, though unseen to the naked eye, expelling our own body wastes and toxic chemicals. Have you ever wondered why, without deodorant, we stink? It's because our bodies are eliminating junk. It's the truth.

The Bible tells us that one day King Saul entered a dark cave "to attend to his needs" (1 Sam. 24:3). Get it? Because porta potties didn't exist in those ancient days, especially in the Judean wilderness, Saul chose a cave as a place to respond to nature's call. While they may seem like the lowliest parts of life, the truth is that daily bowel movements, the process of urination, and even the act of sweating helps keep us clean. In fact, our bodies are the most effective detox aids we've got, and just in case you haven't fully realized it yet—you only have one. If you ruin it, you're sunk. That's why it makes sense to value our bodies (even though they are far from perfect) and to strengthen them through wise choices.

Speaking of detox, this seems like a good time to mention certain foods well-recognized for their purifying effects, such as lemons, grapefruit, garlic, onions, cilantro, plus dark green, leafy vegetables. These all have powerful healing properties that nourish the body and naturally assist its own efforts to eliminate poisons.

Beyond these, here's a few additional detoxification aids I personally believe are worth considering. As I have already shared, my wife Kristin and I honestly believe that the natural product, PCA, developed by Maxam Nutraceutics, and those chelation pills properly prescribed by Dr. Mundall, helped detoxify our son Seth during the height of his battle with seizures. (FYI, I have lab reports in my office from medical doctors demonstrating PCA's ability to increase heavy metal excretion in urine and feces.) Based on my research, another potent purging aid is zeolite powder that can literally suck heavy metals from the body. (Read the published study on www.zeohealth.com.) Activated charcoal is also often used in hospitals and is even recommended by US poison control centers in emergency situations. Used topically or internally (as a drink, mixed with water), charcoal can safely absorb and remove toxins right out of the body. Pharmaceutical-grade bentonite clay works wonders too (as a drink or bath). Charcoal and clay are inexpensive and natural. Used properly by many health warriors worldwide, they can be highly effective in assisting the body's natural efforts to remove killer chemicals from our polluted cells.

Finally, in her heavily-documented book, *Detoxify or Die,* toxicology expert Dr. Sherry Rogers, MD highly recommends infrared saunas for super detoxification through sweating. Our family has one of these saunas. Personally, I love it. A good infrared sauna isn't cheap, but if you can afford one they're worth the price.

Here's one word of caution. Solid science and clinical testing should back up all credible detox aids. So, as I always suggest, do your homework and seek the proof beyond the hype. Paul's counsel is pertinent, "Test all things; hold fast what is good" (1 Thess. 5:21).

Bottom line: The body is capable of detoxifying itself, and sometimes that's all we need. Yet in emergency situations due to severe toxicity when the battle is fierce, certain natural products can assist nature with the purging process. These can be weapons, too, in the fight for our health.

TRUTH: DRUGS DON'T HEAL
DISEASE, NATURE DOES

When sickness strikes, the easiest path is to visit the family doctor, then a pharmacist, and to take a pill. But the truth is (and all soldiers should add this knowledge to their arsenal), *drugs don't cure disease, nature does.* But please don't misunderstand me. I'm not saying there's no place for qualified physicians, pharmacists, and medication, especially in dire situations. Yet prescription drugs are often abused. Now don't miss this point: Generally speaking, most modern medicines merely alleviate symptoms of an underlying problem without touching the primary cause.

To illustrate, imagine that an automobile's check engine light suddenly starts flashing on the dashboard because a serious malfunction has developed under the hood. What should be done? The most sensible solution is to find a qualified mechanic, identify the problem, and fix it. But another option exists. Because the check engine light can become bothersome, a person could just cover those two words with dark tape. "Ah," the foolish soul might say after such a flimsy solution, "the light doesn't bug me anymore."

Would this solve the problem? Hardly. Not only that, but whoever drives that car would risk serious consequences down the road, even a breakdown. It's the same with many prescription medications. Yes, they may relieve acute symptoms of a deep health issue, but the root problem often remains. Even worse, medications often have toxic side effects, which can create even more ills. Worse still, the original problem may become even more serious *while the drugged pill popper doesn't feel a thing.*

Scary thought, isn't it?

Generally speaking, painful symptoms are the body's warning signals that something is wrong and should be corrected. Because this is true, it's perilous to merely suppress nature's merciful sirens, which is what drugs often do, without correcting the underlying problem. If a man's lungs ache because he's addicted to cigarettes, he needs more than a purple pill to mask the pain. Instead, he should quit smoking! If he does, it's amazing how marvelously the human body, the best doctor in town, can heal itself when given the right tools and a reasonable chance.

Remember—nature heals, not drugs.

Truth: Natural Healing Takes Time

Back to plants. Seeds planted in a garden don't produce food overnight. But eventually, after weeding (removing the enemy), watering, and adding proper fertilizers (which provide nutrients plants need to grow), the result is delicious peas, corn, tomatoes, peppers, or broccoli. It's the same with human health. By resolutely removing the choking weeds of nasty habits and by consistently (a key word) replacing them with wholesome ones, eventually, as surely as ripe fruit appears on cultivated vines, we also shall reap a rich harvest of improved health.

But again, this takes time.

Nature works slowly, but surely and wisely.

If you think about it, most worthwhile endeavors take time. Developing good relationships, getting an education, learning a trade, building a house, becoming an athlete, or earning a living all take time, but the rewards are worth it. It's the same with our health. By consistently practicing healthy habits and obeying natural laws, aches and pains can vanish, rashes and sores can clear up, breathing can improve, elasticity increase, bones move more easily, circulation quickens, blood pressure drops, brain fog lifts, and memory once again can become as sharp as a tack. Even cancerous tumors can disintegrate and vanish. *I feel great!* are words spoken by thousands today who, after making diligent efforts to consistently obey natural laws, are reaping the rich rewards of patient persistence in following a healthy lifestyle.

"Rome wasn't built in a day," I often tell Seth. Although Mark Antony, Cleopatra, and Julius Caesar are long dead, that old saying remains true today.

Remember, girding our waists with truth is part of dressing ourselves with "the whole armor of God" (Eph. 6:11). Believe me, all health soldiers need each truth listed above to most effectively fight against killer diseases and win the war, especially in these toxic end times.

Consider what you've learned so far as basic training. Now that you know these facts, you're ready for advanced intelligence information. Prepare yourself. You are about to discover the Big Eight, some of nature's finest weapons for defeating demons who want to kill us.

Chapter 6

EIGHT WEAPONS FOR WINNING THE WAR

The first wealth is health.
—RALPH WALDO EMERSON (1803-1882),
American essayist, lecturer, poet

It's time to unveil eight critical keys to staying alive in these toxic, high-stress, cancer-filled "last days" (see 2 Tim. 3:1) of earth's history. To be clear, I didn't invent these keys. Quite the contrary, they are confirmed by science, understood by knowledgeable doctors (naturopathic and medical doctors), and promoted by health experts worldwide. For further research, Google each item. The facts are there. These keys also represent the backbone of the world-famous NEWSTART program conducted at Weimar Institute in California and operated by Seventh-day Adventists, whom *US News Health* reported to be the longest living people in America.[16] NEWSTART has helped thousands win the battle against heart disease, diabetes, and other lifestyle-related illnesses. The word *NEWSTART* is a clever acronym for:

N = Nutrition
E = Exercise
W = Water
S = Sunshine
T = Temperance
A = Air
R = Rest
T = Trust in God

As you will soon discover, these eight keys—or eight doctors, also often referred to as the Eight Laws of Health—are not only weapons to help prevent killer diseases, but they can often cure them too. Consistently followed, the Big Eight can not only help us win the end times health war, but they can make us feel fantastic. Have you heard the phrase, "keep it simple stupid"? I know you're not stupid, but my point is we all crave simple solutions to life's challenges, especially health challenges. When it comes to the Eight Laws of Health, they're not hard to grasp. Even my kids understand them. You can too. So let me explain these essentials, one by one.

(WEAPON 1) GOOD NUTRITION: EAT MORE REAL FOOD, NOT JUNK

[God] *causes the grass to grow for the cattle, and vegetation for the service of man, that He may bring forth food from the earth* (Psalms 104:14).

After forming man "in His own image" (Gen. 1:27), "The Lord God planted a garden eastward in Eden, and there He put the man whom He had formed" (Gen. 2:8). Think about it. Sinless man's original home wasn't a high-rise apartment or condo inside a smoggy city, but a colorful, pristine, living *garden.* Imagine that! And that garden (called the Garden of Eden) was filled with delicious food created by God Himself for human sustenance and enjoyment. Whether you are a vegetarian or not, the truth is that God originally designed human bodies to be fully nourished by eating a wide variety of colorful, aromatic, super nutritious, and superbly delicious *plant foods.*

"To you it [plant life] *shall be for food*" (Gen. 1:29), declared the Lord to Adam. Today, modern science abundantly confirms God's plan. The facts are in. Eating an abundance of fresh fruits, vegetables, nuts, and seeds, in as simple and natural state as possible, does wonders to build health and counteract disease. One of our biggest problems, even more serious than a sluggish economy and combating Al-Qaeda, is that so much of what enters our mouths and slides into our stomachs is highly refined, heavily processed, genetically modified, and overly saturated with man-made chemicals, preservatives, additives, colorings, flavorings, dyes, heated oils, excessive sugar, and too much salt. From a health standpoint, it's a disaster. Apple-flavored candy isn't good. Applesauce is better. But by far the best of all is to sink one's teeth into a crisp, fresh, ripe apple picked straight off a tree.

"An apple a day keeps the doctor away," reveals a deep truth. Many mysterious health issues are rooted in the simple fact that millions of us keep clogging our cellular machinery with health-destroying garbage. "Life is a tragedy of nutrition," stated health pioneer Arnold Ehret. While it's impossible to take a time machine back to Eden, the more unprocessed and unrefined whole fruits, vegetables, grains, nuts, and seeds we place into our mouths, prepared as simply as possible, the more vitamins, minerals, easy-to-digest proteins, essential fatty acids, cancer-fighting antioxidants, and phytochemicals will pass through our digestive tracts, enter our bloodstreams, and be transported to our cells.

To help you grasp the significance of good nutrition, here is just a small list of only a few of the nutrients derived from food, and just a tiny fraction of their complex functions to protect, enhance, and maintain our health. Many benefits haven't even been discovered yet.

Vitamin A

Essential for cell reproduction and formation of hormones. Helps keep skin, eyes, bones, teeth, and the immune system healthy.

B Vitamins

Involved in RNA and DNA production. Necessary for energy metabolism, forming red blood cells, proper nerve function, and brain health.

Vitamin C

Essential in tissue formation, maintaining cell membranes, for healthy skin, bones, cartilage, blood vessels, and the immune system.

Vitamin E

Plays a major role in protecting and healing body tissues. Protects skin, eyes, and liver. Essential for healthy red blood cells.

Vitamin K

Essential for bone health, regulates blood calcium levels, crucial in the blood clotting process.

Calcium

Essential for building strong bones, blood clotting, enzyme regulation, blood pressure maintenance, and heart health.

Magnesium

Essential for energy production; healthy muscle, nerve, heart and brain function; bone structure; detoxification; and calcium balance.

Iron

Essential component of red blood cells which carry oxygen and nutrition to the rest of the body.

Sodium

Maintains intercellular water levels, pH balance, and normal function of nerves.

Potassium

Maintains the body's fluid balance, blood pressure, heartbeat, nervous system, muscle function, and is essential for proper growth.

Chromium

Necessary for controlling blood sugar levels.

Zinc

Necessary for cell growth, wound healing, and a healthy immune system.

Sound serious? No doubt. I hope this small list convinces you of the critical importance of proper nutrition in the war for our health. Now here's a key point worth stressing: Not only are most highly processed foods nutrient deficient, but all nutrients depend on other nutrients and co-factors to work properly. Thus the ideal way to get vital nutrients, with co-nutrients in their proper ratios, is by eating *real foods*—as God created them—that naturally contain them in proper combinations. It's unimaginably complex, yet simple. Don't miss this: It is by eating more real foods in these end times—which was God's perfect plan at the beginning—that we can best fortify our physical bodies and immune systems to counteract apocalyptic, killer diseases.

On the other hand, modified-by-man, chemically saturated, nutrient depleted, overly salty, sugary, greasy "junk food" stresses, burdens, weakens, debilitates, acidifies, unbalances, and slowly kills the entire system. The wise sayings, "Many dig their graves with their teeth," "The longer the shelf life, the shorter your life," and, "The whiter the bread, the sooner you're dead," sound sober warnings. Personally, if a food product has an unusually long list of ingredients, especially if many of those ingredients are practically unpronounceable, I'd rather avoid it.

But Steve, I just love those tasty foods, you may be thinking. If this is the case, perhaps it's time to do some resisting, don't you think? Seriously, if your taste buds have become addicted to man-altered products so that simple and more wholesome natural cuisine seems unappetizing and boring, my advice is— start slow. Go step by step. Try making just a quarter of your meal more natural. Then half. Or try skipping a meal or two.

You won't die. In a short time, simpler nutritious food will start tasting better. Believe it or not, taste buds can change.

God will help you.

To significantly boost your health, consider consuming more of these well-recognized "super foods" in their natural state: apples, blueberries, bananas, watermelons, tomatoes, lemons, walnuts, kale, broccoli sprouts, cilantro, sunflower seeds, coconuts, garlic, chia seeds, and freshly ground-up flax seeds. Believe me, all of these super foods are bursting with nutrients. If you want to get really aggressive, consider soaking raw nuts before eating them, and even sprouting seeds and whole grains which cause their cancer-fighting nutrient profiles to practically soar off the charts (more on this soon). The bottom line is to eat more real foods as God designed. If we do, our bodies will become stronger and healthier, we'll get sick less, and we'll live longer too (barring unexpected catastrophes).

"Let *food* be your medicine," declared Hippocrates, the father of medicine, "and medicine your food." The old man was right. *Nutritious food is medicinal.*

And never forget this one thing—nature cannot be improved upon.

(Weapon 2) Exercise: We Must Get Off Our Bottoms and Move

Bodily exercise profits... (1 Timothy 4:8).

Have your heard the saying, "Use it or lose it"? It's true. Human bodies were designed for motion, not stagnation. Joining a health club is great, but if this isn't convenient, the most affordable and beneficial option available to everyone is to simply take a daily walk. Studies show that walking even a half hour a day—with your head held high, in the open air, breathing deep—is enormously beneficial. Personally, I like to take a mellow stroll after a meal. It helps digestion and gives my whole body a pleasant boost. Regular exercise also helps the body eliminate deadly toxins and poisonous waste through the kidneys, bowels, lungs, and skin. Why do you think people often stink after a hearty workout? Once again, the reason is simple: they are eliminating junk. So if you want to be healthier, get off the couch and move. It's an established fact. Again, ask your doctor. If he's honest (which most doctors are), he'll probably admit that he needs more exercise too. If you aren't used to it, start slow and then steadily and reasonably increase the pace, whether walking, hiking, biking, or swimming. When I exercise, I feel fabulous!

You can too if you firmly set your mind to it.

(Weapon 3) The Wonders of Water

And He showed me a pure river of water of life, clear as crystal, proceeding from the throne of God and of the Lamb (Revelation 22:1).

But I don't like water, you may be thinking. Perhaps not, but your life literally depends on this tasteless liquid. Approximately 65 to 75 percent of *you* is *water*. You can't live without it. Besides oxygen, water is the second most vital substance needed to sustain life. Your brain, internal organs, ability to digest and assimilate food, blood flow, capacity to eliminate toxins, and even your ability to sleep, jump out of bed, walk, drive a car, or read this book is entirely dependent upon water.

Most Americans don't drink enough water. Instead, too many of us prefer coffee, Coke, or Pepsi. Believe it or not, the following is only a partial list of what simply drinking enough water can do for us:

- Make our muscles more flexible

- Invigorate mind and body

- Sharpen the intellect

- Lower blood pressure

- Remove toxins from the body

- Clear up many bladder problems

- Aid digestion

- Lubricate the body

- Help rebuild cartilage

- Regulate body temperature

- Keep bowel movements regular

- Relieve depression[17]

If you want to improve your health, it's a scientific fact that one of the easiest things you can do for yourself is to just to drink *more water*. The rule of thumb is to drink half your weight in ounces per day. So, if you weigh 150 pounds, your goal should be approximately 75 ounces each day. To make it easier, spend a few bucks and buy yourself a half-gallon water bottle. You may have to visit the bathroom a bit more throughout your day, but isn't that better than riding horizontal beside a paramedic? Many nutritionists also suggest that drinking a glass of warm water mixed with freshly-squeezed lemon juice first thing in the morning does wonders. This simple act helps cleanse, lubricate, and invigorate the entire system. "Water keeps the plumbing humming," is another wise saying.

Again, ask your doctor.

The simple habit of drinking more water could save your life.

(Weapon 4) Let the Sunshine In!

Truly the light is sweet, and it is pleasant for the eyes to behold the sun (Ecclesiastes 11:7).

"Avoid sunlight like the Black Death, or get skin cancer!" the public has been consistently warned since the 1980s. "Not so fast," counters Michael F. Holick, PhD, MD in his eye-opening book, *The Vitamin D Solution*, which explains the critical importance of vitamin D, which our bodies make naturally when sunlight caresses our skin. Professor of medicine, physiology, and biophysics at Boston University Medical Center, Dr. Holick is one of the world's leading vitamin D researchers. Bucking the trend of avoiding an "evil sun" at all costs, Dr. Holick contends that human cells throughout the body have vitamin D receptors, showing sunlight and vitamin D's critical importance. Also, the farther north people live from California, Texas, and Florida, the higher the rates of cancer, cardiovascular disease, and autoimmune diseases they succumb to.

In other words, lack of sunlight *can kill.* Shockingly, Dr. Holick also believes—as do many other vitamin D experts—that the popular "avoid the sun with loads of sunscreen" mantra we've been pounded with since the 1980s is way overblown, has created a dangerously misinformed public "ludicrously fearful of the sun,"[18] and has resulted in untold damage by contributing to widespread vitamin D deficiency—one of the biggest casualties of our time. Except to sunscreen companies, which profit enormously.

Today, vitamin D research is cutting edge and intense, and the current consensus among those who know the facts is that this amazing substance—which the body turns into a hormone starting with direct sunlight falling on unprotected skin—has myriad functions and is absolutely essential for human health. First and foremost, vitamin D helps the small intestine absorb calcium from food. Beyond this, its receptors are found inside brain, breast, heart, pancreas, prostate, colon, and blood vessel cells—even immune system T cells. The Vitamin D Council (a potent resource for more information), founded by Dr. John J. Cannell, MD, reports that only "some of the functions of the body that vitamin D helps with include":

- Immune system, which helps you to fight infection

- Muscle function

- Cardiovascular function, for a healthy heart and circulation

- Respiratory system—for healthy lungs and airways

- Brain development

- Anti-cancer effects[19]

This makes Doctor Sunlight pretty important, don't you think? The primary caution with sunlight exposure is to avoid burning the skin. If we get regular, proper amounts of sunlight but not too much to damage our skin, Dr. Holick contends that the risk of malignant skin cancer is minimal or non-existent. If you live in northern latitudes (like my family does in north Idaho), Dr. Holick also strongly suggests: 1) that you get your blood vitamin D level tested with a 25-hydroxy vitamin D test to know if you are deficient or not, and 2) if you are deficient, that you take inexpensive vitamin D supplements (and/or use a sunlamp like the vitamin D lamp, model D/UV-F manufactured by Sperti) until your blood serum levels rise to normal.

So what's normal? The debate is ongoing, but many vitamin D-savvy doctors, experts, and researchers now suggest an optimal level of between 50 to 100 ng/ml (nanograms per milliliter). As of this writing, the Vitamin D Council suggests 50 ng/ml as "ideal." Others shoot for 80 to 90 ng/ml. Regardless, both the Vitamin D Council and Dr. Holick strongly contend that tragically large numbers of us are vitamin D deficient, don't even know it, and suffer for it. Dr. Holick even calls vitamin D deficiency "the most common nutritional deficiency in the world"[20] that has now reached epidemic proportions.

Another valuable book is *The Vitamin D Revolution* by Dr. Soram Khalsa, MD. Clinical professor of medicine and past chairman of the advisory committee for the

Environmental Medicine Center of Excellence at Southwest College of Naturopathic Medicine in Tempe, Arizona, Dr. Khalsa strongly concurs with both Dr. Holick and the Vitamin D Council. Surprisingly, Dr. Khalsa even reports, "In a review of 18 different vitamin D deficiency studies, it was found that people taking vitamin D were *less likely* to die from any cause while people not taking vitamin D supplements were *more likely* to die."[21]

Amazing. This again highlights not only the value of direct sunlight, but even the life-and-death potency of vitamin D supplements if enough sunlight isn't available in your area. Now, here's something else of interest about our son Seth. As of this writing, Seth has taken no anti-seizure medicine for over four years. Thankfully, he's doing great. Nevertheless—and this has been a mystery to my family— for the last few years he has developed a pattern of having a small cluster of short seizures in November/December. Then, they stop. Last year it was the same thing. In 2013, this happened in the month of November *only*. As we discussed this with our family physician, Dr. Angelika Kraus, she had a new thought. "Perhaps it's vitamin D related," she suggested.

Upon reflection, her theory makes sense. We live in north Idaho, and each fall as the days get shorter and the sun drifts farther away, Seth has a cluster of short seizures. Then each December our family flies south to warmer climates to visit relatives or take a vacation; each time we do, Seth's seizures cease. We recently tested Seth's vitamin D blood levels, and he was on the low side. So, at Dr. Kraus' recommendation, we've bumped up his supplementation to

5,000 IUs of D3 daily (most researchers recommend D3). Our goal is to get his blood levels to around 80 ng/ml. We'll see what happens next year. If this theory is correct, this suggests that both heavy metals and lack of sunshine are co-culprits in Seth's condition. Ultimately, only God knows all the causes, but we are doing our best to figure it out.

Here's another quick tip. Getting your D levels tested by your family doctor can be a bit pricy. If finances are a factor, cheaper options exist online. The Vitamin D Council's website recommends the ZRT vitamin D home test kit for 65 dollars. Or shop around. Wherever you go, be sure to request a 25-hydroxy vitamin D test. Dr. Khalsa also recommends making sure the lab that reads the blood sample has a certificate from DEQAS, the Vitamin D External Quality Assessment Scheme.

The bottom line is that if you have the luxury of living in a warm climate with lots of sunlight, *don't let the devil keep you in the dark.* If you don't have that luxury, get as much sunshine as reasonably possible and then supplement appropriately if necessary. In light of the fierce controversy between God and Satan, it makes sense that in these end times the Prince of Darkness would craftily seek to keep humans away from sunlight's healing rays—under the guise of protecting our skin from skin cancer—as a strategic weapon of mass destruction.

As the lyrics of a once-popular song recommend, "Let the sunshine in!"

You will be a lot healthier if you do.

(Weapon 5) Temperance

The fruit of the Spirit is love, joy, peace, longsuffering, kindness, goodness, faithfulness, gentleness, self-control (Galatians 5:22-23).

To be blunt, most of us eat far too much food. The phrase "I'm stuffed" says it all. We call this *overeating*. The Bible calls it *gluttony* (see Prov. 23:2,20-21). The current epidemic is more serious than we realize. Not only are rates of obesity soaring even among children, but so are killer diseases that accompany extra pounds around waistlines. "I want it when I want it, and I want it now," is the language of this generation. If we know what's good for us, we'll resist such craziness and fight for our health. "Eat less, live longer," is another wise saying. "Caloric restriction means longevity," is a technical way of saying the same thing. This definitely holds true for rats in a lab, and it's true for humans too.

The overall idea is called "temperance," which includes self-control. Unfortunately, it's nearly a lost art. Essentially, to practice temperance means to be moderate in the use of what is good and to abstain from what is harmful. I know it's not easy to resist temptation and conquer bad habits, but don't forget this is war and our enemy is *targeting our taste buds*. If we're going to survive in these end times, we have to buck the current, swim upstream, and take a stand, which many times means to shut our mouths and avoid consuming harmful things.

Again, the facts are in. The evidence is overwhelming that consuming alcohol slowly destroys liver function, tobacco and nicotine cause lung cancer, caffeine overstimulates the brain and nerves, excess fat clogs arteries leading to high blood pressure and heart disease, and too much sugar weakens the immune system. The true path to health, or to its recovery once we've lost it, is to develop a firm and consistent habit of saying "No!" to unhealthy substances that are slowly killing us, no matter how aromatic, popular, tantalizingly delicious, or seductive they may be.

"Just say no to drugs," is a common slogan.

To win the war against our health, saying *no* applies to more poisons than heroin.

(WEAPON 6) FRESH AIR: OXYGENATE YOUR BODY

The Lord God formed man of the dust of the ground, and breathed into his nostrils the breath of life; and man became a living being (Genesis 2:7).

Air. It's even more vital than water and food. We can survive for weeks without food, days without water, but only a few minutes without oxygen. Air enters our lungs when we breathe, is miraculously transferred to trillions of red blood cells in our bloodstreams, and is then pumped by the heart to waiting cells throughout our bodies, from head to toe. Each cell needs oxygen to function efficiently. Without oxygen, living cells weaken, degenerate, suffer, and die. Or they mutate, become sinister (almost with minds of their own) and even cancerous. To be healthy, we must keep our cells healthy with plenty of oxygen. Then they remain "good guys," instead of being transformed into malignant, militant mutations.

Come on, everybody breathes, you may be thinking, *so what's the big deal?* Yes, we all inhale and exhale, but many critical factors influence the amount of oxygen that reaches our cells. One big factor is diet. Eating lots of "bad fats" can make the bloodstream thick and sluggish, which results in less oxygen reaching cells. Alcohol also causes red blood cells to clump together, causing similar problems. Failing to drink enough water makes blood thicker too. Cigarette smoke clogs the lungs with black goop, lessening the amount of oxygen that reaches the bloodstream. So does inhaling secondhand smoke from smokers or even just breathing polluted city air. Indoor air too, if windows are never opened, becomes stale and devitalized.

Here are some tips. Stop smoking. Forsake alcohol. Drink more water. Get outside as much as you can. Exercise in the open air. Open windows in your home, office, and car more often. Finally, practice deep breathing from the diaphragm (lower chest) instead of from the top of the lungs. Many articles exist online about the positive health effects of regular, deep breathing. It's relaxing, alleviates stress, soothes the nerves, and increases overall oxygenation throughout the body. In a nutshell, oxygen means life. Its lack causes death. Make no mistake about it, the battle for pure air is a big part of the Great War.

So open the windows and let Doctor Air flow in.

And guess what? He'll never send you a bill.

(Weapon 7) Rest: Don't Burn the Midnight Oil

I will both lie down in peace, and sleep; for You alone, O Lord, make me dwell in safety (Psalms 4:8).

We all need rest and sleep, generally between seven to nine hours per night. The habit of staying up late will slowly but surely take its toll, weakening the entire system. Sleep experts warn us that if we regularly deprive ourselves of necessary ZZZs, we'll pay the piper sooner or later. The whole body will suffer, and we will reap sickness. Maybe even death. Sleep experts also contend that every hour of sleep before midnight is worth two after midnight. I believe it.

In our home with our two children, as a general rule, it's lights out by 8:00 p.m. My wife and I usually join the kids between 9:00 and 10:00 p.m. For me, it wasn't always that way. During my childhood years, I often watched television past midnight. In my late teens, there were many nights when I stayed out until the wee morning hours with the guys. But now all has changed. During those wild days, I once spied a slogan on a bathroom wall stating, "He who hoots with the owls at night can't soar with the eagles in the morning." To this day, I haven't forgotten that slogan.

In his article, "Top 10 Health Benefits of a Good Night's Sleep," Mark Stibich, PhD references clinical evidence showing that regular sleep boosts heart health and memory, reduces cancer risk, lessens stress and inflammation, and allows the body necessary time for rebuilding and repair.[22] If you eat an evening meal, it's best to finish it a few hours before retiring so that you go to bed on an empty stomach. If undigested food requires processing during the night, the body has extra work to do, which detracts from what it needs to do most—rest, detoxify, and rebuild.

So don't eat late, and go to bed earlier.

In April of 2012, CBS News (quoting the CDC) warned that over 40 million Americans are sleep deprived. Not only that but the sleep industry, which now offers an almost endless variety of how-to-get-your-ZZZs gizmos, is *a 32 billion dollar business*.[23] While some sleep disorders may be unavoidable, if we will only obey natural laws more carefully we can save big bucks and sleep better too.

Isn't it time that we *wake up* to our need for a better night's sleep?

As with all the Eight Doctors, getting enough sleep is another critical weapon we must wield in the raging war for our health.

(Weapon 8) Trust in God: The Moral Factor

Trust in the Lord…depart from evil. It will be health to your flesh, and strength to your bones (Proverbs 3:5,7-8).

"Be pure. It's what doctors recommend most." How often have you heard this during a television commercial? Yet it's the truth. Deep within each human head is a mysterious something called the *conscience*, which somebody once defined as "that little part of us that feels awful when the rest of us feels great!" When we yield to temptation, commit a sin, or do what we know is wrong, we experience guilt. Our moral violation may be hidden from the eyes of friends, co-workers, relatives, or even a spouse, but deep inside *we know what we did*. Although many doctors often ignore this basic principle, the fact is that a prolonged sense of guiltiness is 100 percent disease producing.

The Bible says, "Trust in the Lord...depart from evil. *It will be health to your flesh, and strength to your bones*" (Prov. 3:5,7-8). Did you catch that? Trusting in the Lord and renouncing evil brings health. As a pastor, husband, and father, I now realize this as never before. When I believe in God's steadfast love, repent of my sins, trust my Savior's mercy and forgiveness, and then through His power live a morally pure life, the result is not only that my conscience becomes clean, but I feel better too. Seventh-day Adventist health educator Ellen G. White wrote insightfully:

> The consciousness of right doing is the best medicine for diseased bodies and minds.[24]

She was right. Morality and health are inseparable. Our sin-sick world may not grasp it, physicians may not take courses about it at Harvard or UCLA medical schools, nor pharmacists prescribe it, but daily doses of faith in God and obedience to the Ten Commandments promote peace of mind and exert healing influences upon the central nervous system. According to the Holy Bible, our struggle against sin itself is at the heart of the Great War. And sin not only endangers the soul, but it damages the body too.

"A merry heart does good, *like medicine*" (Prov. 17:22), says the Good Book. It's the truth. A happy heart, a pure conscience, high morals, and vibrant health all fit together like a lock and a key. That's why "Trust in God: The Moral Factor" is the capstone of the Big Eight. To reject this is catastrophic.

Take A Step

At this point, you may feel a bit overwhelmed by the thought of so many changes you may need to make in your life. If so, I understand completely. Here are two tips. First, remember this old Chinese proverb, "The journey of a thousand miles begins with a single step." Second, the good news is that you don't have to face your foes alone. "I am the Lord who heals you" (Exod. 15:26), says our merciful Creator to each one of us as long as we are willing to do our part and begin the journey. But once again, don't forget that we are at war with more than flu bugs. The Devil is no wimp, and cancer kills. If we refuse to fight and just go with the flow, eventually we may receive an unexpected, dismal diagnosis.

So don't give up. "I will strengthen you, yes, I will help you," says the Lord (Isa. 41:10). For our encouragement, King David also wrote, "In the day when I cried out, you answered me, and made me bold with strength in my soul" (Ps. 138:3). Paul also testified, "I can do all things through Christ who strengthens me" (Phil. 4:13).

That's it for the Big Eight. Before this book is over I'll give you a few extra arrows in your quiver to rout the enemy.

Chapter 7

SPECIAL FORCES: FRESH, RAW JUICES

...drink the pure blood of the grape
(Deuteronomy 32:14 KJV).

Have you heard the news? Purchasing a juicer; squeezing fresh juices from raw carrots, beets, celery, kale, lemons, apples, and grapes; and "juice fasting" have gone mainstream. Why is this? The reasons are simple. People are tired of feeling miserable and are trying to reboot their health—naturally, by themselves, in the privacy of their own homes. Millions also wish to avoid expensive trips to medical offices, ERs, and hospitals in addition to bypassing surgery, chemotherapy, and radiation treatments, all of which are not only traumatic on the body, but can also decimate a hard-earned bank account. Helpless dependence on medications isn't fun either, especially if better options exist.

Another reason for the juice revolution is that scientific studies are now confirming what countless health enthusiasts have already experienced—*the life-changing, healing power of unprocessed, freshly squeezed raw juices.*

Before noting some of these scientific studies, the American Cancer Society has already gone on record stressing the critical importance of upping one's daily intake of fruits and vegetables. Beneath the headline, "Add Fruits and Veggies to Your Diet," the official ACS website declares:

> Eating lots of fruits and vegetables can help reduce your cancer risk. That's one reason the American Cancer Society recommends eating at least 2½ cups of these foods every day.[25]

Thus, even the ACS has served us notice that consuming larger amounts of fruits and vegetables can "lower cancer risk" and save lives. So what about their juices? Can they be life-saving as well? You are about to find out.

One of the most unstoppable forces fueling today's explosively popular juicing movement is the inspiring story of Australian businessman Joe Cross as told in his self-produced documentary, *Fat, Sick & Nearly Dead*, which won first place as Best Documentary Feature at the Iowa Independent Film Festival in 2010. The summary on the movie's website declares:

> A hundred pounds overweight, loaded up on steroids, and suffering from a debilitating autoimmune disease, Joe Cross is at the end of his rope and the end of his hope. In the mirror he saw a 310-pound man whose gut was bigger than a beach ball and a path laid out before him that wouldn't end well—with one foot already in the grave, the other wasn't far behind.

Fat, Sick & Nearly Dead is an inspiring film that chronicles Joe's personal mission to regain his health. With doctors and conventional medicines unable to help long term, Joe turns to the only option left—the body's ability to heal itself. …Joe finally trades in the junk food and hits the road with juicer and generator in tow, vowing only to drink fresh fruit and vegetable juice for the next 60 days. Across 3,000 miles Joe has one goal in mind—to get off his pills and achieve a balanced lifestyle.[26]

Wow! A 60-day juice fast! Did it work? Watch the DVD. It will make you cry. *Yes, it did.* Joe had help too. Dr. Joel Fuhrman, MD, author of *Fasting and Eating for Health: A Medical Doctor's Program for Conquering Disease,* oversaw Joe's journey step by step, taking blood tests and monitoring Joe's heart. Mr. Cross shed his excess weight, kicked all his meds, and got his life back. Today, Joe's story has inspired millions to take their own juice plunge. "Sales of juice extractors are soaring," is the excited testimony of juice machine makers like Breville (used by Joe Cross in the movie), Omega, Jack Lalanne, and Lexen.

If you do a search on Amazon.com for books about juicing and juice fasting, you'll find titles like *Juice Fasting for Detoxification: Using the Healing Power of Fresh Juice to Feel Young and Look Great* by Steve Meyerowitz, *Juice Fasting for Weight Loss* by Kamal and R. Kishore, *Juicing Recipes* by Drew Canole, and *The Juicing Bible* by Pat Crocker. There's even *The Complete Idiot's Guide to Juicing*, written by the founding food editor of *USA Today*, Ellen Brown, and *Juicing and Smoothies for Dummies* by Pat Crocker. Don't miss the significance of these last two titles. Whenever "Idiot's Guide" and "Dummy" books hit bookstores, you know a major trend has captured public interest.

Now for some well-researched facts. Dr. Michael Greger, MD runs the website, www.nutritionfacts.org dedicated to establishing a scientific basis for his belief that a totally vegetarian, plant-based diet is truly optimal for human health. A founding member of the prestigious American College of Lifestyle Medicine, Dr. Greger is licensed as a general practitioner specializing in clinical nutrition. His website declares:

> Dr. Greger scours the world of nutrition-related research, as published in scientific journals, and brings that information to you in short, easy to understand video segments.[27]

Dr. Greger is quite a detective, and in video after video he provides compelling evidence that whole, unaltered, unprocessed fruits, vegetables, whole grains, beans, nuts, seeds, roots, and select herbs have remarkable healing powers. In conjunction with a healthy lifestyle, Dr. Greger establishes that the regular consumption of these foods—in their natural state—has almost miraculous powers to renew, revitalize, and regenerate human cells, fight cancer, counteract chronic diseases, boost energy, and make a person feel great!

So we ask again—what about the juices of raw plant foods? Might they have super-concentrated nutrition?

Here's Dr. Greger's answer, using kale juice as an example.

In his video presentation, "Smoking Versus Kale Juice," Dr. Greger first quoted that "Kale juice has gained increasing attention as one of the popular health-promoting foods in

Japan." Based on the published results of a Japanese study, he then reported:

> Thirty-two men with high cholesterol consumed three or four shots of kale juice a day for three months. That's like eating a total of 30 pounds of kale, the amount the average American consumes in a century. What happened? Did they turn green, start to photosynthesize? What it did was dramatically lower their bad cholesterol and boosted their good cholesterol as much as would an hour of daily exercise seven days a week. Obviously, by the end of three months the antioxidant level of their blood shot up significantly.[28]

Dr. Greger's position is, by all means, eat kale and plenty of it. But if you want to supercharge kale's positive effects on your cholesterol and antioxidant levels, *then drink kale juice.*

As with kale, so with beets reports another peer-reviewed article published by The Journal of American Physiology entitled "Acute and Chronic Effects of Dietary Nitrate Supplementation on Blood Pressure and the Physiological Responses to Moderate-intensity and Incremental Exercise." This scientific study analyzed the effects of "supplementation with beetroot juice" for "4-6 days" in "eight healthy subjects." In a few days, drinking that juice was shown to acutely reduce blood pressure and improve exercise tolerance.[29] This study helps to explain the rapid lowering of my own blood pressure during my three-week juice fast described earlier. I juiced lots of beets. (Note: Don't worry, I haven't forgotten to finish that story. I'll return to it in the next chapter.)

One treasured book in my library is called *Becoming Raw* by Brenda Davis, RD; Vesanto Melina, MS, RD; and Rynn Berry. What I appreciate most about this book is that it examines the nutrient content of plants from a scientific standpoint. (FYI, I still eat what I consider to be a reasonable amount of cooked food.) Past chair of the Vegetarian Nutrition Dietetic Practice Group of the American Dietetic Association, Brenda Davis and her co-authors have done their homework. Citing peer-reviewed scientific research from sources like *The American Journal of Clinical Nutrition*, *The International Journal of Food Science Technology*, and *The Institute of Medicine*, one key paragraph in *Becoming Raw* declares:

> Some carotenoids—such as alpha-carotene, beta-carotene, and lutein—appear to be more bioavailable from vegetable juice than from raw or cooked vegetables [references cited]. Women who consumed vegetable juice had almost three times the alpha-carotene and 50 percent more lutein in their blood than others who consume the same amount of these carotenoids from raw or cooked vegetables [references cited]. …Juicing, pureeing, other otherwise breaking a food down into smaller particles enhances the bioavailability of phytochemicals [references cited]. In addition, juicing removes a good portion of the plants cell walls and membranes, reducing fiber and other compounds that can inhibit the absorption of nutrients and phytochemicals.[30]

Yes, science definitely does support juice power.
Because of this, I believe the juice revolution is here to stay.

The basic philosophy behind juicing is that the combination of living on a toxic planet tainted with heavy metals, DDT, PCBs, and Agent Orange residues, harmful habits (think coffee, alcohol, and cigarettes), plus the regular intake by most Americans of hundreds of pounds of processed, devitalized, chemically-saturated junk foods is slowly killing us. As a result, human cells are sick, and we need to make major lifestyle changes in order to win the war for our health. In the process of trying to recover health or to protect it once we have it, guess what can give us an extra boost? You got it—freshly squeezed, raw juices.

Let me clarify some things. First, I'm not talking about store-bought juices. Yes, they can provide some benefit, but heated, pasteurized apple, orange or grape juice doesn't compare to fresh juice. Second, I'm also not suggesting anyone subsist solely on raw juices (although you probably could if necessary), but rather that freshly squeezed raw juices can be *a key auxiliary weapon* in cooperation with a healthy lifestyle which should already include good nutrition, plenty of pure water, exercise, moderate sunlight, fresh air, and proper amounts of sleep.

Dr. Thomas Lodi, MD declares that raw plant juices contain "mega amounts of nutritional substances" that are invaluable "for renewal and regeneration."[31] Dr. Lodi is no novice. From 1991 to 1996, he served as Clinical Instructor of Medicine at the University of Hawaii School of Medicine, and he is the founder of an alternative cancer treatment center called "An Oasis of Healing" located in Mesa, Arizona. Inside the book *The Complete Idiot's Guide to Juice Fasting* by Steven

Prussack and Bo Rinaldi, in a chapter called "Stories of Transformation," Dr. Lodi offers this amazing report:

> A fellow from the west coast came to our center with stage-4 lung cancer, which carries an extremely dismal prognosis. He drank four to five quarts per day of fresh, green vegetable juice, and within five weeks a PET scan was unable to detect any active cancer. The same has occurred with stage-4 pancreatic cancer, as well as every other cancer, albeit in differing amounts of time. Of course, this is not all they were doing, but those who don't happily and gratefully do a juice fast do not get these results. The same rate and depth of healing occurs with all other chronic diseases such as diabetes, high blood pressure, arthritis, digestive malfunctions, and others.[32]

Isn't that encouraging? Yes, even cancer can be beaten, and raw juices are valuable weapons to help win the war.

Join the revolution. Get a juicer.

So much for technicalities. Let's get practical. So what do you do? First, yes, you can use a blender, which is great, especially for fruit smoothies. But if you really want to experience the full benefits of freshly squeezed juices, they should ideally flow from a quality juice extractor specifically designed to remove fiber (more on this soon) and maximize nutrition. Thus, the best thing is to do some research and invest in a juicer. "If you don't have one, buy one today. It will save your life," wrote the famous herbalist Dr. Richard Schulze in his popular book, *There are No Incurable Diseases*.[33]

Which juicer should you buy? Honestly, this isn't the easiest question. But don't worry, here's some tips. A good place to start is by visiting http://discountjuicers.com/juicers.html run by juice expert John Kohler. I appreciate John; he has lots of energy, and his simple videos are quite informative about the pros and cons of different models. Last I checked, his YouTube channel had nearly seven million views. In considering which juicer to purchase, the main factors to consider are:

1. Size

2. Weight

3. Ease of use

4. How dry is the pulp?

5. Amount of juice you get

6. How much foam?

7. How much nutrition is preserved?

8. Durability

9. How noisy is it?

10. Your family size

11. Customer service

12. Reviews

13. Price

14. The warranty

Only you can decide which factors are most important to you.

After doing my own research and watching Mr. Kohler, I decided to purchase an Omega 8004 (about 250 dollars) for my home. This unit is sturdy, single augur, rotates slowly (creating hardly any heat thus preserving more nutrition), leaves dry pulp, produces little foam, and is super easy to clean (between one and two minutes). Believe me, the easy-to-clean factor is huge, because practically speaking, the majority of juicers that aren't usually end up gathering dust. The Omega 8004 also has a fabulous 15-year warranty.

Of course, you have options. Mr. Cross used a Breville model in *Fat, Sick & Nearly Dead,* and Jack LaLanne juicers are popular, both of which cost a bit less than the Omega 8004. Then there's the little manual "Healthy Juicer" by Lexen for under 50 dollars which is primarily designed for juicing leafy greens, sprouts, microgreens, and above all, wheatgrass (more on this soon). Once you visit John Kohler's website and pick a model to consider, I suggest you visit YouTube.com, type in the name of that juicer, and look for videos discussing the pros and cons of that model. Finally, read the customer reviews on Amazon.com. Then make an informed choice.

Next, obviously you need something to juice. During my three-week fast—and still today—I juiced lots of carrots, beets, celery, lemons, limes, and a few apples to sweeten my cup. If you are diabetic, you should avoid juicing too many fruits, because the concentrated sugar content could raise your blood sugar a bit. Of course, if you have any major health challenges, you should always consult your health care provider for guidance. If your doctor knows nothing about the benefits of juicing, either kindly suggest that he or she get with the times and read up, or find another doctor who does. With all the scientific studies being conducted these days about the incredible health benefits of raw plant juices, there's really no excuse not to know about it.

If you have a garden, this is the best place to start. This way you can get fresh, organic produce without chemical fertilizers, pesticides, herbicides, and fungicides, which is always best. If not, go to the produce department of your local market. If you can afford it and if they have it, buy organic. If not, my advice is to load up anyway. From my research I have concluded that it is better to juice commercially grown produce than not to juice at all. You will still get loads of benefits. Plus, as your body gets healthier it can more effectively detoxify itself of poisons. But if you don't want to take any chances, then by all means buy only organic. Costco often carries 25-pound bags of organic carrots at a good price. Or try Wal-Mart.

Juice experts generally recommend choosing many varieties of plants. To boost the health benefits, juice lots of *green leafy vegetables* rich in chlorophyll which help purify the blood, increase oxygenation, alkalinize the body, and detoxify the liver. Watermelons are terrific too, rind and all. Same with lemons. Sweet peppers and grapes add a pleasant taste. An internet search for "delicious juicing recipes" will yield lots of results. The list is endless. My advice is— don't limit yourself. Add variety. Experiment. Increase your weapons. You'll get more nutrients to fortify your system to fight disease.

PRACTICAL DETAILS: WHAT TO DO

I like to juice first thing in the morning, drinking my fresh elixir right away, on an empty stomach, about a half hour or so before breakfast. The quicker you consume what flows from your machine the more nutrients you get, because the longer juice sits the more oxidation occurs. With the Omega 8004, clean-up is so easy, so you can juice what you need, drink it immediately, clean up, and then put the juicer away until your next session. Another option is to juice more than you need and then pour the extra juice into glass jars for storage in your refrigerator for later. Fill those jars to the brim (to minimize oxidation), seal them tight, and then drink up within 24 to 48 hours.

When I juice, the first thing I do is get set up. Out comes the juicer. Then all produce is placed in the sink for a reasonable washing. Certain veggies are then placed onto a cutting board so that, based on the size of my juicer's chute, they can be cut with a knife to fit. Beets, lemons, and apples are cut into smaller pieces. Harder apples juice better. Fatter, larger carrots get sliced up, while thinner ones, along with celery stalks, stay right in the sink until they go straight down the chute. For softer produce like tomatoes or grapes, it is best to alternate between harder produce and softer. Things flow better that way. Dedicated citrus juicers are also available.

I typically drink between eight to twelve ounces at a time. That's enough until next time, which could be later in the day, usually about an hour before lunch or an hour before supper. Personally, I don't drink with my meals, for I don't think this is best for digestion.

About fiber. Fiber is vital because it acts like a broom in the digestive tract to keep food flowing through the body so our plumbing doesn't get clogged. Fiber is essential for health for a host of reasons and helps prevent colon cancer. Significantly, fiber, which is indigestible, is found only in plants. Meat and dairy products have none. I don't juice for fiber, but for extra nutrition. So I try to remove all the fiber, that way when the juice enters the body it is most easily digested and assimilated without the body having to perform much work.

One simple thing to do is to go to a hardware store and buy a small nylon meshed bag used for thinning paint. They cost about one dollar each. Right before my three-week juice fast in the summer of 2012 I bought one, and I am still using it today. When fresh juice comes out of my Omega 8004, I always strain that juice even further by pouring it carefully through the mesh into another, separate glass or container. Then, down the hatch. Nice! Again, I don't juice for fiber (I get plenty of fiber in my regular meals), but for mega amounts of vitamins, minerals, enzymes, cancer fighting antioxidants, phytochemicals, and for whatever else science hasn't discovered yet. Think about it. Eating ten carrots is great, but it will take you quite a while to chew and swallow them. Through the miracle of juicing you can insert ten carrots into your juicer and quickly drink all their nutrients in a glass or two, thus getting the nutrition of ten carrots in a fraction of the time.

Not a bad deal, don't you think?

If you aren't a juicer expert, no problem. The main thing is to start juicing. Veggie after veggie, cup after cup, session after session, you'll start feeling the difference. If you make mistakes, no biggie. Just juice! You'll learn as you go.

SHORT AND LONG JUICE FASTS

About fasting. Generally speaking, fasting is another incredible weapon against disease that we should be wielding in these end times. But, in contrast to juicing (which is easy), fasting is trickier and requires more training. First, I recommend you read up a bit on both the benefits and risks (there aren't many, as long as you follow common sense) of either juice or water fasting.

Essentially, to *fast* means to avoid solid food for a time. Juice fasting is easier than water fasting, so if you want to fast I recommend a juice fast first. To get your feet wet, try skipping just one meal and replacing it with juice. Next, skip two meals. Then three. Most people can easily handle skipping solid food for one to three days and juicing instead. If you have some extra pounds to shed, this is a perfect place to start. One benefit of juice fasting, in contrast to water fasting, is that it is less stressful on the body. With juice, you still get calories, energy, and fabulous nutrition. Short juice fasts shouldn't interrupt your normal schedule either. You can still go to work, exercise, etc.

The point is to start slow. After trying the above for a bit, you might try avoiding solid food one day a week for a month or two. Then, if you wish, try advancing to two days per week for another month. Again, no solid food, just juice. Believe it or not, growing numbers of health-conscious housewives, blue-collar workers, and white-collar professionals are experimenting with such things right now around the world, and they are experiencing incredible benefits. Again, most people can easily handle all such beginner juice fasts without serious problems.

For longer fasts, I strongly recommend connecting with an expert, such as a knowledgeable medical doctor, credible naturopathic doctor, or other health professional who knows about juicing. Believe it or not, their numbers are growing too. *Therapeutic fasting* is the term now being used by fasting-informed doctors like Dr. Joel Fuhrman, MD; Dr. Thomas Lodi, MD; and many others who regularly fast their patients with serious health challenges.

On the other hand—and all fasters should mentally prepare for this—there will be days when the faster will feel totally drained, with no pep at all. Zero. At those times, one should rest. No exercise. Nothing. But those periods of weakness generally don't last long, and then strength returns. Fasting experts sometimes call these uncomfortable episodes part of a "healing crisis." The idea is that when you cease eating solid food for a time—which takes lots of energy and inner resources to digest—while at the same time flooding your cells with mega-nutrition by drinking fresh-squeezed, raw, no-fiber juices, your body finally has time to wisely attend to something else. Detox. Cleansing. Housecleaning.

To further illustrate, imagine a mother who is so busy cooking in the kitchen for a family of five that she hardly has time to take out the trash. So, garbage builds up. The stench grows. Eventually, family members get sick. *Stop the show!* the mother realizes. Then she takes a break from cooking for a day or two to clean up the mess. It's the same with our bodies. Day after day, week after week, month after month, year after year, we eat, eat, and eat, and much of this food is hard to digest (such as high-protein animal products, or even highly-processed vegetarian food that may be loaded with chemical additives and heated oils). Yes, we do eliminate much of this waste regularly through our bladders, bowels, skin, and lungs, but because our systems are normally so preoccupied with handling food, they often don't have enough time or energy to remove *all* of the trash. So garbage builds up, which is then stored in various organs and fat cells. Eventually, we get sick. Or worse still, deathly sick.

At that point, we risk losing the war entirely. But when a person counterattacks by fasting (avoiding food) and drinking raw juices, the body's innate artillery revives. Complex hormones are produced, and war signals are then sent to cellular DNA with the message, "Activate the troops. Mobilize and eliminate garbage." When this happens, watch out. Boils, headaches, fevers, or massive mucous elimination may result, and we can feel weak, tired, or even worse, very ill. But don't worry. The body has the situation under control. Normally, in time these battles will pass. After our enemies are driven out, we will feel better than ever.

In *The Complete Idiot's Guide to Juice Fasting,* in that chapter referred to earlier called "Stories of Transformation," is another almost unbelievable account from a man simply listed as "Steve." Here is his report:

> I was in my late 30s, working as an occupational therapist with autistic children. I decided to start juicing for a few days. I wasn't sure how long I was going to fast; I just knew I wanted to drop the extra fat around my belly and hopefully get my cholesterol down. My body went into a major healing crisis and started pouring years of accumulated junk out of my body.

The most profound thing happened. I had given up smoking more than fifteen years before this cleanse and exercised just about every day. Yet one morning I noticed the tips of my fingers were starting to peel. I looked closer, and saw black soot coming out of the tips of my fingers! I inspected the soot, smelled it, and found it was actually nicotine coming out of my body! It was stored in my fat cells and finally was being released thanks to a raw food diet and juice fast![34]

Can you believe it? Many others can testify of similar experiences after juice fasting, water fasting, or even from just abandoning junk food, giving up animal products, eating more raw plant foods, drinking more water, and stepping up their exercise routine. As to the power of juicing itself, here are four more stirring testimonials I discovered in the "customer reviews" section for the Omega 8004 juicer on Amazon.com:

I have bought it [an Omega 8004 juicer] a year ago and believe me it will change your life. I am a 26-year-old guy, work out five days a week, and was very healthy till last year. I was having persistent headaches and dizziness all of a sudden. I have been to many doctors including specialists (neurosurgeon, ENT) but nothing was diagnosed in any of my tests. So I thought of vegetable juices, and believe me it worked. It took more than three months but it healed. I have bought two more machines, one for my parents and [the] other for my sister's family. This is the best gift you can give to your family.

—RAVI[35]

In the past few months of using this model about twice a day, with plenty of greens like wheatgrass (growing my own on my balcony), kale, collards, parsley... mixed with mostly carrots and also apple and celery, my enlarged prostate problem has disappeared!

—ALBERT VALENTINO[36]

My wife had multiple stomach and duodenal ulcers from medications due to a spinal injury and we combed the internet looking for studies on the best home remedies, as prescription antacids were not healing her. We chanced across two studies on raw cabbage juice healing ulcers in a matter of weeks, so that led me to research juicers. ...We've now used it [the Omega 8004] more than 60 days on cabbage and broccoli. ...My wife's ulcers completely healed by the two month point, so we've moved on to juicing other items.

—AARON[37]

First let me tell you that my life has changed since I began juicing. I am in my mid-thirties and I felt like a 60-year-old person with a lot of health issues. Since I began juicing most of my health issues have gone. I lost 30 pounds [and] I feel like a person my real age or younger. My skin has changed. When I see in the mirror and I see literally a younger person. My wife says I have rejuvenated. Even though I am older than my wife she says I look younger than her. Juicing vegetables is the real fountain of "eternal" youth.

—MR. PERFECTIONIST[38]

Isn't that marvelous?! Again, juicing really works.

Essentially, freshly squeezed, raw plant juices are God's special forces to pump super nutrition into our fantastically organized bodies so they can drive out inner invaders, rejuvenate our cells, zap cancer cells and tumors, repair damaged DNA, fight disease, and help us win the war for our health.

Ready, aim, fire! has become my motto.

Chapter 8

STRUGGLES, DISCOVERIES, VICTORIES

If there is no struggle, there is no progress.
—FREDERICK DOUGLASS (1817-1895),
African-American social reformer

Back to my battle. It was June 23, 2012. In disbelief, I stared at my blood pressure monitor—196 over 76. "You need to get back on the meds right away!" a tempting voice seemed to relentlessly urge inside in my head. *Oh, what shall I do?* During the past week, which was the first week of my juice fast, my blood pressure had steadily dropped, down to as low as 110 over 63. That very morning, I had abandoned my blood pressure medication for the first time in five months, hoping my problem was whipped forever. Now this. Should I retreat back to those drugs or advance forward?

The battle was on. To me, it felt like life or death.

"I'm going for a walk," I quietly informed my wife and some friends who were visiting at our house, then I slipped out the back door. Totally downcast, I headed for the back end of our property nestled on the edge of an Idaho forest. Out in the woods, surrounded by towering ponderosa pines and red firs, I dropped to my knees before my Maker and breathed out three simple, heartfelt requests. First, that I wouldn't die. Second, that God would help me to stay off the medications, which by that time I had become fully convinced were not a healthy permanent solution and possibly quite harmful. Third, I asked Him to heal me fully and bring my blood pressure down.

It was a frightful moment. Remember, I have a family to support. Yet deep in my soul I just knew that retreat wasn't the answer, and so I leaned heavily on the Lord to hear my prayer and have mercy upon me. After perhaps twenty minutes of prayer and pleading, I slowly walked back to my family and friends.

The answer to my first request is obvious. I'm not dead yet. Second, I've been medication-free since that very day, and I have firmly decided that I am definitely not going back. Third, have I been healed? Keep reading.

The next day I phoned Linda Clark and explained my dire situation. To me, her response was life-changing and part of God's answer to my prayer. Since I took my blood pressure reading the day before, my mind had mainly focused on that upper, systolic number, 196 (remember, 120 is normal). In the midst of my mental confusion, that was all I could see. "Think about the lower number, Steve," Linda countered, "It's perfect. This tells me you are making real progress."

These words were like a bright ray of heavenly sunlight flashing into the midst of one of my darkest hours. *Hmm...* "You're right!" I replied, as the truth sank in.

"Stick with the program," Linda continued. "Your body will heal itself, but it takes time."

In retrospect, I'm not sure whether that 196 reading was a withdrawal symptom of getting off the medication or if it was my diseased condition viscously fighting back against three of God's most powerful natural remedies: 1) pure water, 2) potent herbs, 3) nutrient-loaded raw, fresh plant juices. Or it may have been a combination of all three. But one thing I do know: My struggle was intense. It was a battle within, and my body felt like a war zone.

I won't go back, I finally informed my invisible foes. *No chance.* So I forged ahead, continued my fast for two more weeks, ended with three days of eating nothing but fresh fruit, and then returned to my deepening commitment of trying to eat more natural foods, exercising more, drinking lots of pure water, and trying my best to obey nature's laws. In the days that followed, sure enough, the good days increased, and the difficult days decreased. Now, there's one thing I want to state clearly to every reader of this book, and it is this—healing doesn't come overnight, that's for sure, and I had plenty of ups and downs. Remember, nature works slowly, and natural healing takes time. But if we stick with our decision to obey nature's laws, positive results will finally come just as surely as God Himself still reigns upon His throne.

Here's another experience worth noting. Most of the time fasting experts recommend plenty of rest during times of no solid food, with little physical activity, so Dr. Body can focus its attention on what it does best—routing enemies and healing what ails us. Nevertheless, each of us is unique, and we must often forge our own path. In my case, during my fast, yes, there were days when I felt rotten with no energy. Zero. Zip. Then, I rested. But on other days, my energy level soared. As you know, I like to jog. Now, I've never run any marathons (and never will), but four to five miles at a slow, steady pace feels great. I especially like to run up logging roads in the forest near our house with our dog, Pooka. During my three-week fast, I was surprised to find myself going farther and farther, higher and still higher up those hills.

Like I said, fresh juice plus lots of water really works.

Here's something else. About a month after my fast, which took place in late June/early July of 2012, another amazing thing happened. In August, I didn't feel sick or have a cold, but for three solid weeks I coughed up, hacked up, or sneezed up more mucous than in my entire life (or so it seemed). It was phenomenal. After my sinuses normalized, a new thought struck me forcibly. *Wow*, I thought to myself, *a month ago I flooded my system with super nutrition for three weeks. Now I just finished another three-week period of massive mucous removal.*

More house cleaning, I concluded.

To me, everything fit. Three weeks of God's nutrients, then a month where my immune system was gearing up for another calculated assault on my diseased condition, and then three weeks of purging. Nutrients in. DNA notified. Weapons sequence initiated. More bad guys out. After that particular immune system surge was over, I felt even better!

During my June/July journey, I decided to post some details on my Facebook page. As a result, I received lots of responses and questions from a whole host of cyber buddies. "I want to do a juice fast too," some said. "What do I do?" At the time, I certainly felt like no expert (I'm still not, but I've learned a lot), but those pleas touched my heart. Eventually, they compelled me to action, which is one reason why I wrote this book.

August slipped into October. Then on October 12, 2012, I visited an ENT (ear, nose, and throat) specialist in Spokane, Washington for an unrelated nasal issue. Unexpectedly, a nurse slipped a blood pressure band around my right arm. "A hundred ten over sixty-three," she said. "You have the cardio-vascular system of a twenty-year-old." I could have kissed her! (I didn't.) At that instant I knew once again, as I continue to realize today, that *God answered my prayer in the Idaho forest.* "He delivers me from my enemies," wrote King David in Psalms 18:48. I feel the same too. Praise His name!

As I write this, it's now June, 2014. I am still medica-tion-free, and thankfully, most of the time I feel really good. "Today is a good day," I heard a preacher once say. "Any day above ground is a good day!" Whatever daily ups and downs come my way, I concur wholeheartedly with that preacher.

Before closing this chapter, there are a few more lessons I want to relay. In the heat of my high blood pressure battle, I happened to be reading the book *Counsels on Health,* which is a compilation of the insightful health writings of Ellen G. White. My eyes fell upon these words:

> Satan is the originator of disease, and the physician is
> warring against his work and power.[39]

I lowered the book, paused, pondered, and then reread that sentence. Finally, its impact sank in. *I'm fighting the devil,* I solemnly realized. What a revelation. It's the truth. Whether we realize it or not, all disease, from the common cold to cancer, is to some extent and in some mysterious way the work of Lucifer himself and a sign of his "power." Think with me. Before Adam bit the forbidden fruit, he was 100 percent healthy; after he rebelled against God, it's been downhill ever since. Therefore, in the light of the big biblical picture, all sin and sickness come from Satan. He is the *ultimate destroyer* of human health—the invisible impulse behind all bodily break-downs. According to the Holy Bible, he hates God and you and me. He wants us all dead. But when we renounce him and his evil ways, trust the Lord, and then make wise, healthier choices, we are fighting back against the devil's legions. Notice carefully what the Scripture says:

> *When the sun was setting, all those who had any that were sick with various diseases brought them to Him [to Jesus]; and He laid His hands on every one of them and healed them. And demons also came out of many, crying out and saying, "You are the Christ, the Son of God!"* (Luke 4:40-41)

Thus when Jesus healed people of "various diseases," "demons also" were forcibly expelled from human bodies. This shows a mysterious relationship between disease and devils. In another instance, Jesus encountered "a woman who had a spirit of infirmity eighteen years, and was bent over and could in no way raise herself up" (Luke 13:11). Like I said, I'm not a doctor, but from what I've read this sure looks like a classic case of a medical condition known today as *kyphosis*. Whatever her exact disease, notice carefully how the Bible says that beneath this woman's woe was "a spirit of infirmity." When Jesus healed her, "she was made straight, and glorified

God" (Luke 13:13). Now here's a key point. After a misguided religious leader complained that Jesus had performed this miracle "on the Sabbath" (Luke 13:14), the Master countered His accuser with, "ought not this woman, being a daughter of Abraham, whom *Satan has bound*—think of it—for eighteen years, be loosed from this bond on the Sabbath?" (Luke 13:16).

Did you catch that? Perhaps this poor lady did have kyphosis or arthritis or osteoporosis, but underneath her real physical illness *Jesus detected a satanic influence.* "Whom Satan has bound" was His heavenly diagnosis. Once again, this shows that the devil is behind disease and suffering. Yes, diseases may (and do) have natural causes, but there are supernatural influences too. If this is true (which it is), then to most effectively combat sickness, we should recognize the influence of both and seek God's help. Ultimately, all disease is the fruit of sin, and whether God chooses to heal instantly (which He sometimes does, as in Bible days) or more slowly through the weaponry of our immune systems which He carefully created, all genuine healing is a merciful, miraculous manifestation of God's vastly superior strength working against Satan's own "work and power."

If you think about it, this makes perfect sense. Doesn't the immune system itself manifest intelligence? No doubt. It is extraordinarily sophisticated, far beyond our complete comprehension. God is behind it, for He created it. It's the same with disease. Mysteriously, sickness has dark, intelligent components. Colds and flu bugs *strike*. Viruses *attack*. Osteoporosis *depletes* bones. High blood pressure *beats* against internal organs. Neurodegenerative diseases *slowly destroy* the brain. Mutant cancer cells stealthily *maneuver* around sophisticated immune defenses. Some metastasize and recruit more cells. Once they've gathered an army, they march for the kill.

Do you grasp what I'm telling you? Again, this is war. When we're sick, dark forces seek strongholds. Our immune systems fight back, but disease fights back too, fueled by hosts of darkness. Even when we make wise choices, sometimes things get worse before they get better, because unseen foes viciously resist our healing. At the height of my high blood pressure conflict, I felt like I was being ripped apart. But God helped me. In my case, He didn't heal immediately, yet He worked steadily through my juice fast. Nutrients flooded my system. Cellular troops rallied. Victories were gained. Personally, I now believe my condition stemmed from a combination of depleting vital nutrients (such as magnesium) due to stress, overtaxing my brain, and decreasing levels of vitamin D due to living in northern Idaho—all fiendishly influenced by devilish foes. There may be additional factors I haven't realized yet. Honestly, I'm still learning. But now I believe for sure not only that an ancient enemy was involved in my difficulties, but also that the Lord God of heaven and earth Himself counteracted with His power and did wonders in my life. Whatever your situation, He will help you too if you pray earnestly, trust Him, seek to understand the root causes of your ailments, and then determine to fight back by more fully obeying His health laws, all of which were established for our happiness.

Just to clarify again—I certainly can't guarantee that every disease will vanish from our bodies in this life, even if we do everything right. It may or may not. In my struggles, I've also learned the valuable lesson that God often uses sickness and suffering as wake-up calls—to drive us to Him, to correct bad habits, to purify our hearts from sin, and to lead us to focus on eternity. Truly, He's a skillful expert at bringing blessings out of curses. Case in point: Because of Seth's seizure battle and my own conflict with high blood pressure, I have discovered so much, and this has led me to write this book, which hopefully will help you too. I've also learned that whatever our case, conflicts, cares, confusion, or condition, "the sufferings of this present time are not worthy to be compared with the glory which shall be revealed in us" (Rom. 8:18).

I'll explain more about that "glory" before this book is done. But before that, I'll share one more powerful weapon against the Disease Originator.

It's called *live* food.

So turn the page.

Chapter 9

MORE SPECIAL FORCES: SPROUT POWER

And God said, "See, I have given you every herb that yields seed which is on the face of all the earth, and every tree whose fruit yields seed; to you it shall be for food" (Genesis 1:29).

"Due to economic considerations," a farmer told me recently, "I spray Roundup on my fields four times a year. I used to spray only once."

Hmm, I thought to myself, *this can't be good.* Why not? Isn't Roundup safe? Monsanto claims so, millions think so, and Roundup is daily sprayed around the world onto crops humans regularly eat. Yet consider this: in June of 2009, an Environmental Health News article reported:

> University of Pittsburg ecologists added Roundup at the manufacturer's recommended dose to ponds filled with frog and toad tadpoles. When they returned

two weeks later, they found that 50 to 100 percent of the populations of several species of tadpoles had been killed.[40]

Thus, Monsanto's popular herbicide—even "at the manufacturer's recommended dose"—can terminate more than weeds. But shouldn't it be safe for everything else? Ask those dead tadpoles. Brace yourself. It gets much worse. To start with, the same *Environmental Health News* article also stated that "researchers have found that one of Roundup's inert ingredients can kill human cells" too.[41] And that's just *one* ingredient. So for me, no matter what Monsanto's highly paid toxicologists claim about the safety of their product, I'd like to keep their chemicals out of my body as much as possible.

Looking at the big picture, here's a scary fact: "Approximately 5.1 billion pounds of pesticides are used each year in the United States," stated the US Environmental Protection Agency in May of 2012.[42] That's an awful lot of chemicals being sprayed on our food. I realize that farmers regularly use and handle them, but don't miss this: many often wear full body protection gear as they do. Why such protection? One reason is because containers holding such chemicals often state in bold letters, "Danger—harmful or fatal if inhaled, swallowed, or absorbed through the skin." If that's not enough of a reason, the *skull and crossbones images placed beside those warnings serve as added incentives*. Yet, even after precautions are taken, the National Cancer Institute still recognized that:

> General studies of people with high exposures to pesticides, such as farmers, pesticide applicators, manufacturers, and crop dusters, have found high

rates of blood and lymphatic system cancers; cancers of the lip, stomach, lung, brain, and prostate; as well as melanoma and other skin cancers.[43]

Driving one last nail into the coffin of listless indifference to the threat of chemically saturated crops, the 2008-2009 Annual Report of the President's Cancer Panel recommended eating "food grown without pesticides or chemical fertilizers" to reduce cancer risk.[44]

Thus, after reviewing the hard data, even the President's Cancer Panel has warned Americans to eat foods grown "without pesticides." All of this should make it painfully obvious that serious health risks *do* exist, not merely from largely-void-of-nutrition snacks and processed foods, but even from near-perfect-looking fruits and veggies sold at grocery stores (which, by the way, are still much healthier than junk food). It's because of these factors, plus deepening anti-GMO concerns (read the book *Seeds of Deception* by Jeffrey M. Smith), that more and more Average Joes like you and me are planting their own gardens and growing their own food. It's why the term *organic* has become a household word.

Yet maintaining a home garden takes substantial time and effort, and most of us don't own enough land to even attempt to start one even if we wanted to. Now listen carefully. If your own health and that of your loved ones is truly important to you (if it isn't, you need serious enlightenment), and if space, cost, and time are scarce, guess what? I have more life-saving information for you. I'm about to teach you how to grow your own extra-nutritious, anti-cancer, anti-heart disease, pesticide-free *live food* at little cost, inside your own home, year-round (even in winter), all the while making allowance for your busy schedule.

Sound too good to be true?

It's not.

Keep reading.

TEN REASONS TO SPROUT

Welcome to the exciting world of sprouting burst-ing-with-nutrition, tiny plants from seeds and growing them in small jars and trays. In his bestselling book, *Sprouts, the Miracle Food: The Complete Guide to Sprouting*, Steve Mey-erowitz, a.k.a. "The Sproutman," lists these "10 Reasons to Start Sprouting!"

1. ECONOMICS Seeds can multiply 7-15 times their weight. At $4.00/lb. for seed, that yields 26 cents for a pound of fresh, sprouted, in-door-grown organic greens!

2. NUTRITION Sprouts are baby plants in their prime. At this stage of their growth, they have a greater concentration of proteins, vitamins and minerals, enzymes, RNA, DNA, bio-flavo-noids, T-cells, etc. than at any other point in the plant's life—even when compared with the ma-ture vegetable!

3. ORGANIC No chemicals, fumigants, or ques-tions about certification. You can trust it's pure because you are the grower!

4. AVAILABILITY From Florida to Alaska, in January or July, enjoy live food anytime, anywhere, even on a boat or when hiking a mountain trail.

5. SPACE-TIME It's easy! Just add water! No soil. No bugs. No green thumb required. No special lights. One pound grows in only 9 inches of space and takes 1 minute of care per day.

6. FRESHNESS Because they are picked the same day they are eaten, there is no loss of nutrients sitting in crates or on grocery store shelves.

7. DIGESTIBILITY Because sprouts are baby plants, their delicate cell walls release live nourishment easily. Their nutrients exist in elemental form...mak[ing] them easy to digest even for those with weak digestion.

8. VERSATILITY More varieties of salad greens than on your supermarket shelves—including buckwheat lettuce, baby sunflower, French onion, garlic chive, Chinese cabbage, purple turnip, curly kale, daikon radish, crimson clover, golden alfalfa and more. Your salads will never be boring again!

9. MEALS Make sprout breads from sprouted wheat, rye, or barley. Snacks from sprouted peanuts, hummus dip from sprouted garbanzo, cooked vegetable side dishes made from sprouted

green peas, Chinese sauces from mung, adzuki, and lentils—even sprouted wheat pizza!

10. ECOLOGY No airplanes or fuel/oil consumed to deliver the food to you. No petroleum-based pesticides or synthetic fertilizers.[45]

The Magic of Seeds

Before zeroing in on details, consider the incredible power of seeds. Believe it or not, all life on planet Earth is dependent on these mysterious, miniature miracles. First, all plants come from seeds. Without plants, which produce oxygen, there wouldn't be enough air for humans to breathe, and we would all quickly perish. Even if you aren't a vegetarian, you still eat some plants, and even the animals you consume receive their core nutrition from plants, which spring from seeds.

Get it? Without seeds we're done, extinct, non-existent.

Next, seeds also have incredible *longevity*. When Egyptologist Harold Carter discovered King Tut's tomb in 1922, bean seeds were found there too. Later, they were soaked in water, and guess what? They sprouted after lying dormant for nearly 3,000 years! The same can never be said about any cow, fish, bird, or meat product.

Beyond longevity (seeds can survive far longer than any animal or human now living), seeds are extremely *powerful*. Not long ago I was jogging on a narrow, concrete path in rural Michigan. Glancing down, I was amazed at the sight of small mounds that looked like miniature volcanoes popping up along the path. What caused those two-inch upheavals?

Answer: sprouting seeds, weighing a mere fraction of the weight of the concrete they literally busted up.

Science can never fully explain the mystery. When seeds receive water and begin to germinate underground, the small plants develop terrific pressures capable of shifting dirt and rocks and cracking objects far heavier than their own weight. Stories have even been told about sailing ships literally splitting asunder when rice seeds in the ships' cargo holds became saturated by incoming water and sprouted. Grain silos have also ruptured when too much moisture reached seeds stored inside. In time, growing plants can destroy sidewalks, towering stone statues, and rock walls.

Seeds are phenomenal.

Guess what else? When consumed in their whole, unprocessed, and natural state, seeds are also packed with large payloads of vitamins, minerals, trace minerals, proteins, simple sugars, essential fatty acids, and a whole host of cancer-fighting phytochemicals that can substantially boost your health.

That's not all. Don't miss this. When seeds sprout, the germination process produces major microscopic multiplications of their already fabulous nutritional profiles. "The Sprout-man" reports:

> When sprouting, a seed unfolds and starts to multiply and develop its nutrients in order to provide nourishment for the maturing vegetable. ...Proteins, vitamins, enzymes, minerals and trace minerals multiply from 300 to 1200 percent.[46]

In *Becoming Raw* (referred to earlier), Brenda Davis, RD also cites clinical studies from medical journals confirming that "sprouts provide spectacular amounts of the antioxidant vitamins...[which are] far more effective than using supplements."[47] In other words, if you want to protect yourself from killer diseases and supercharge your health, consuming living sprouts is vastly superior to popping purple pills or even organic green ones for that matter. In fact, live sprouts are some of the most nutritious foods humans can eat.

Those miniature powerhouses are tough to beat. Why is this? The real reason is because, as the Holy Bible says in Genesis 1:29 (quoted at the beginning of this chapter), living seeds and the plants that spring from them were created at the beginning of time by God Himself as the original food for humans.

That's why.

Our Creator knows what's best.

HEALTH BENEFITS OF EATING SPROUTS

In her article, "Composition and Health Benefits of Sprouts," Nita Mukherjee lists these large perks from regularly consuming such small edibles:

- The vitamins and proteins in sprouts help to build muscles and tone the body. Calcium strengthens the bones, while iron boosts the hemoglobin, necessary for transporting oxygen to all parts of the body.

- Sprouts reduce the incidence of cancers, heart diseases and diabetes. They lower cholesterol, and regulate the absorption of glucose from the digestive system. Moreover, they contribute to the health of the liver, spleen and lungs.

- Sprouts increase vitality, strengthen the immune system, detoxify the body and slow the aging process.

- The fiber provides roughage, thus preventing constipation, hemorrhoids and peptic ulcer.

- Finally, sprouts maintain the acid-alkaline balance of the body.

Sprouts are full of vitamins, and easy to digest. They are filling, yet low in calories, thus helping to regulate weight. They rarely cause allergic reactions, and are easy to consume. Crisp, tasty and crunchy, they are a nutritious addition to a number of dishes like salads, soups, sandwiches and vegetable dishes. Sprouts have the highest level of nutrients which are easily absorbed. Therefore, regular consumption of sprouts leads to a heightened feeling of health, energy and vitality.[48]

These facts help explain why, in addition to the global juicing movement, the worldwide sprouting movement has become unstoppable; why Amazon.com contains so many how-to-sprout books; why commercial greenhouses are growing them; why supermarkets now offer them in produce sections; why restaurants and buffets have added them to their menus; why mail order companies deliver them fresh to your door; why scientists are studying them; and why places like

The Living Foods Institute in Georgia are using them to help terminal cancer patients at death's door not only to outwit the Grim Reaper, but also to thrive with new life.

Sprout power is waiting for *you*, too.

Next, I'll show you what to do.

How to Grow Your Own Live Sprouts

The first thing is to get set up. You will need: 1) a jar, 2) seeds, preferably organic, and 3) water. Pretty simple so far, right? Of course, there are many ways to sprout seeds, but one of the simplest methods is with a jar. Glass is best, but not necessary. Almost any container will do. It should have a wide enough mouth to easily pour seeds and water into and to remove your growing sprouts at harvest time. One-quart or half-gallon canning jars are ideal. If you need help with supplies, everything necessary can be ordered from www.handypantry.com or by calling 866-948-4727.

Next, seeds. For beginners, some of the easiest seeds to sprout are larger beans (legumes) like lentils, mung, peas, and garbanzos (chickpeas). Handy Pantry's "Crunchy Lentils Fest Mix," "Bean Salad Mix," and "Protein Powerhouse Mix" contain exciting combinations. Even if your thumb isn't green, it's hard to mess up with these. You'll love them.

Before bedtime, place a few handfuls (one to two cups) of these larger seeds into a jar. Rinse once. Then fill the jar with twice as much water as you have seeds, so your seeds are completely covered with lots of room to swell. Don't worry. They won't drown. Instead, a miracle will begin. Then stick the jar in a cabinet (or anywhere really) for the night.

While you sleep, they awaken. By morning, you will notice that much of the water has been absorbed by the seeds, which may have doubled or tripled in size. Drain the water (don't drink it, although your houseplants will love it), rinse again, and then let them sit (without any water in the jar) until evening. Repeat the same process (rinse again, draining out the water) morning and evening for three to four days, and presto! Your sprouts will grow in the jar until you have a bountiful batch of them.

When their tiny "tails" (roots) are between one quarter to one inch long (based on your preference), rinse thoroughly, add your choice of seasoning, and they are ready for salads, sandwiches, or soups. It's that simple. Add lemon and some garlic to garbanzo sprouts, whip them up in a blender, and you have homemade hummus. No DDT, PCBs, or Roundup—just nature's goodness.

For larger seeds (lentils, peas, garbanzos, mung, wheat, rye, etc.) you can easily use a common household strainer to prevent your seeds from spilling into the sink during rinsing, or you can order convenient Sprout Lids with small holes from Handy Pantry. As an alternative to the jar method, another wonderful and easy option is the highly popular three-tray sprout garden, which works great with either small or large seeds. Simply soak your seeds first in a jar; then transfer them to one, two, or all three trays, which conveniently stack on top of each other.

During the early stages, sprouts prefer darkness (remember, seeds normally start growing underground), which makes them stronger. This isn't necessary though. They'll still grow anywhere. If you are using a jar, place it under a sink, in a closet, or in a cabinet. With a sprout garden, the lids shut out the light. Rinse two or three times a day.

In three or four days, the larger seeds are ready for their new home—*you*. For smaller seeds (alfalfa, clover, or broccoli) let them grow for a while, remove the lids, and then place them in indirect sunlight to green them up (making them chlorophyll-rich). When they look ready, transfer them to your digestive system to supercharge your health. You can also green up smaller seeds in jars too. After three or four days, when leaves appear, set the jar on a windowsill and allow sunlight to do the rest.

If you are concerned about harmful bacteria on seeds (you are more likely to meet your demise in a plane crash than have a problem here), a few drops of grapefruit seed extract (available at www.wheatgrasskits.com or call 866-948-4727) added to your initial soak water should disable any hostile invaders. Room temperature is best. In cold rooms, sprouts grow slower. In hot or humid rooms, they can develop mold or rot. Ventilation helps. If your sprouts stink, trash them. You may need to purchase better seeds.

Hulled buckwheat seeds (called "groats") also sprout wonderfully and only need 20 minutes of soaking (compared to all night). With these, I usually place them inside a colander in a sink after their first 20-minute activation in a jar. As usual, rinse them morning and evening. After two or three days, tiny tails appear. They're ready to eat. I love buckwheat groat sprouts as a morning cereal. They have a pleasant, nutty taste. Add some raisins, bananas, honey, or maple syrup and some rice or almond milk (available at most markets) and you have just made a batch of *living* breakfast cereal that is much healthier than anything in the cereal aisle.

Wheat, barley, and rye (grain) seeds work the same as morning cereals. Raw, hulled sunflower seeds do too. Soak hulled sunflower seeds overnight, grow for two or three days only, then eat as cereal, like buckwheat groats. Trust me. They are far superior to anything you can purchase in a box. Once your sprouts are ready, eat some right away and store the rest in your refrigerator. Eat within three to five days. True grains (wheat, rye, barley, spelt) are easy to sprout, highly nutritious, and can be used in sprouted bread recipes.

Varieties are endless, and there are lots of possibilities at Handy Pantry. Initial soak times may vary too, so check with Handy Pantry or Google each seed. Type "soak time for broccoli sprouts," etc. You'll get the hang of it quickly and learn as you go. Handy Pantry's basic sprout growing kit is a nice option and contains exact instructions. Once you've mastered the simple art of growing sprouts in jars or trays (like a sprout garden), you might consider advancing to microgreens. Some crops take more work, but they are worth the effort.

MARVELOUS MICROGREENS

"Good things come in small packages."

—OLD PROVERB

The colorful book *Microgreens: How to Grow Nature's Own Superfood* by Fionna Hill is priceless. Living in an apartment in Auckland, New Zealand, Fionna has become an internationally recognized microgreen expert. The beautiful (and mouthwatering) photos in her book are absolutely stunning. The basic difference between tiny sprouts and microgreens is that microgreens are grown a bit longer, usually in pots or trays, until their roots are firmly established and tiny leaves develop. After exposure to indoor sunlight—*snip, snip*, into salads they go.

Technically, any sprout that develops leaves and is exposed to sunlight becomes a microgreen (even in jars or a sprout garden), but serious growers normally grow bigger crops in larger trays, often on soil. For everything you need plus free instructional videos, visit www.growingmicrogreens.com or call 866-948-4727 (affiliated with Handy Pantry).

Here's a precious pearl of information. When researchers examined the stages of an edible plant's life—from seed to tiny sprout to microgreen to full maturity—guess which stage packed the most potent nutritional punch? You guessed it— the microgreen stage.

Microgreens Pack Nutritional Punch

"Tiny Microgreens Packed with Nutrients: Microgreens Have Up to 40 Times More Vital Nutrients Than Mature Plants," flashed the headline of a fascinating article published by WebMD Health News. Here's the report:

> They may be tiny, but a new study shows trendy microgreens punch well above their weight when it comes to nutrition.
>
> Researchers found microgreens like red cabbage, cilantro, and radish contain up to 40 times higher levels of vital nutrients than their mature counterparts.
>
> Microgreens are young seedlings of edible vegetables and herbs harvested less than 14 days after germination. They are usually about 1-3 inches long and

come in a rainbow of colors, which has made them popular in recent years as garnishes with chefs.

Although nutritional claims about microgreens abound on the Internet, this study is the first scientific evaluation of their nutritional content. Researchers say they were astonished by the results.

"The microgreens were four- to 40-fold more concentrated with nutrients than their mature counterparts," says researcher Qin Wang, PhD, assistant professor at the University of Maryland in College Park. "When we first got the results we had to rush to double and triple check them."

For example, red cabbage microgreens had 40 times more vitamin E and six times more vitamin C than mature red cabbage. Cilantro microgreens had three times more beta-carotene than mature cilantro.

Researchers evaluated levels of four groups of vital nutrients, including vitamin K, vitamin C, vitamin E, lutein, and beta-carotene, in 25 different commercially grown microgreens.

The results are published in the Journal of Agricultural and Food Chemistry.

Vitamin C, vitamin K, and vitamin E levels were highest among red cabbage, garnet amaranth, and green daikon radish microgreens.

Cilantro microgreens were richest in terms of lutein and beta-carotene.

"All of these nutrients are extremely important for skin, eyes, and fighting cancer and have all sorts of benefits associated with them," says researcher Gene Lester, PhD, of the USDA.

Lester said he was surprised to find microgreens were superior in nutritional value than the mature plants.

"To find that the levels were not only detectible but in some cases 4-6 times more concentrated than in the leaves of a mature plant, I find that quite astonishing."

Although more research is needed, Wang says there may be a good explanation for microgreens' high nutrient content.

"Because microgreens are harvested right after germination, all the nutrients they need to grow are there," says Wang. "If they are harvested at the right time they are very concentrated with nutrients, and the flavor and texture is also good."[49]

Impressive, don't you agree? Once again, seeds, colors, flavors, and textures are endless. Options include alfalfa, broccoli, basil, buckwheat, Chinese cabbage, red clover, yellow mustard, onion, peas, pak choi, radish, and sunflower. Essentially, you need: 1) seeds, 2) a tray, 3) soil or other "growing medium," and 4) water. It's not rocket science, but there's a definite learning curve. Regular growers expect a few failed crops (a minor matter, it happens with sprouts too) and press on.

Any shallow tray, pot, or pan will do, but serious growers often use common 11 by 21-inch seed-starting trays from garden stores or www.growingmicrogreens.com. Many use about an inch of soil (from their yards, local nursery, Wal-Mart, etc.), although the folks at www.growingmicrogreens.com successfully grow microgreens without soil (hydroponically) with "Sure to Grow Pads" as a growing medium where the baby plants take root. Using this method, place one Sure to Grow Pad inside one 11 by 21-inch tray. Add about two cups of water, with a touch of lemon juice (micros love slightly acidic water, 5.5 to 6 pH). Soak the pad well; then sprinkle the dry seeds densely, but just one layer, across the damp pad. Then use a spray bottle to moisten the seeds. Note: for even better results—this applies to all sprouts, initial soak water, misting, etc.—hydroponic microgreen growers often add extra nutrition like liquid kelp or Ionique Liquid Fertilizer (www. handypantry.com) to their water or spray bottles. Then perch a second tray on top of the seed tray, creating a blackout, humidity dome. Remember, sprouts grow best in the dark.

Remove the dome once or twice a day, and keep misting with a spray bottle for three to four days. Your goal is moist, not drenched. Once the plants are fully rooted into the pad (or soil), turn the top tray over and place it directly on the plants so they will become stronger pushing up the tray. A couple of days later, remove the dome, and expose to indoor sunlight. Stop misting now, but water *under* the plants by gently lifting the pad and adding just enough water (one to two cups) to keep the bottom of the pad moist. Or, just water thoroughly at one corner of the tray from a faucet, then drain. After 10 to 12 days, depending on the seed sown, they're ready. Gently cut with scissors close to the bottom of the plants, wash, and eat.

Bon appetit.

Using the above tray method (which also works with a sprout garden), some easy seeds for beginners are broccoli and red cabbage. Sunflower greens are superb, pleasant tasting (*even my kids love them*), and super healthy but trickier, and do best in about an inch of soil in trays. Personally, I have recently been growing a lot of sunflower greens (my children call them "sunnys"). First I soak them overnight, then sprout them for about three days in a jar, then transfer them (not too thickly) onto about an inch of soil in a tray without holes. I water moderately, then cover with a second upside-down tray that rests directly on the plants, with some weight on it (sunflower seeds like the pressure). I usually then check them once a day and mist them if they look a bit dry, doing this for two or three more days. Once the plants are well rooted, I water from the sides and drain thoroughly. After four to five days, I remove the weight (which they have pushed up quite a bit) and then green them up in indirect sunlight. After the plants are tall enough and most of their black shells have fallen off, it's salad time. Believe me, they're awesome. Again, free instructional videos are available at www.growingmicrogreens.com.

Soil or no soil, to supercharge your body, health, and immune system with fabulous nutrition, nothing beats regularly eating *live microgreens*. Growing them is not that hard. And again, you'll learn as you go. Try it. You'll like it.

THE KING OF NUTRIENT THERAPY: WHEATGRASS JUICE

"If I had only one product to give to a patient, it would be wheatgrass." —EDWARD BROWN, MD

Have you heard of wheatgrass? If not, it's time you did. Wheatgrass is actually a microgreen that is super easy to grow in your home from wheat seeds. Before I explain details, read these inspiring testimonies taken from a chapter called "Real Stories from Real People" in Steve Meyerowitz's bestselling book, *Wheatgrass: Nature's Finest Medicine*.

Bladder Cancer

> What can I say? I'm supposed to be dead according to them. My bladder was totally covered with tumors. Now, my MRI doesn't show any. None. My bladder was cut so many times and lasered and scraped and fried. Then the chemotherapy, the radiation, all the drugs. It was awful. It fried the surface of my bladder. And during the whole time, whenever I would go back for an examination, there would always be another tumor or two. ...My daughter from Germany got me started on wheatgrass. ...With her help, I started drinking wheatgrass every day. ...It's been four years now. ...My MRI and sonogram are clean. My bladder is not a problem anymore. My doctor— he's nice, but strictly conventional—says, "Just keep doing what you're doing."
>
> —DOROTHY NAYLOR, Naples, Florida

Breast Cancer

> On March 1 of 1996 I had a needle biopsy which, when the results came in, confirmed breast cancer. My doctor recommended an immediate radical mastectomy and a full program of chemotherapy and

radiation. I'm a registered nurse...so I am well aware of the effects of cancer and the results of treatment. But I just could not go through with it. ...My colleagues were mortified. ...I would never steer anyone away from conventional treatment if that's what they chose. ...But for me, I just could not go through with it. Philosophically, I feel it's the wrong approach—destroying all the good cells along with the cancer cells. I want to strengthen my immune system, not debilitate it. ...So, I was recommended to a holistic doctor...he worked closely with me in developing a nutritional program that included wheatgrass, raw vegetable juices, supplements, exercise, and detox. ...I juiced everything—lots of greens, lots of garlic, sprouts—mostly organic veggies except when I couldn't get them. Most of my friends...are physicians and nurses and at first they told me, "You're in denial," but now they're hushed. ...Since I started the wheatgrass I have more energy than when I was cheerleading in high school! ...I had an AMASS test six months ago and it came up negative. No sign of cancer anywhere! ...I just wish I could sneak a juicer into the hospital and make wheatgrass for all my patients.

—ANNE-MARIE BAKER, Ft. Myers, Florida

Candidiasis, Irritable Bowel, Leaky Gut Syndrome

My problems started during my wrestling years. ...I developed candidiasis, leaky gut syndrome and eventually arthritis. ...I've been fighting this fight for 20 years, now. I've tried everything; nothing works.

Only wheatgrass has helped me. ...Since I've been doing wheatgrass, my digestion is ten times better. My hair got thicker, the white spots left my nails, and the dark rings around my eyes cleared up and the pain in my legs is gone. There is a change in my muscle quality, too. They're firmer; my knees last much longer. ...My candida and my digestion are 100 percent better. I sleep better at night, too....

—TONY GENTILE, Malaga, NJ,
former collegiate wrestler

Colon, Lymph, and Liver Cancer

Gary had colon cancer and six lymph cancers and one spot on the liver. Dr. Botonay heavily insisted on chemo and radiation. I asked him, "If we did all that, would we get rid of the cancer?" He said it would give Gary six more months. Gary and I left his office determined to seek alternatives. ...I'm an X-ray technician and Mom is a nurse. ...[After learning about wheatgrass] Dr. Smith [cancer surgeon] permitted us to give 2 oz. of wheatgrass every 4 hours through a tube in his nose that went directly into his small intestine. My son Kenny and I grew it, juiced it, and gave it to him. Every day we watched his platelet count rise. ...They took blood work up every day. It's fully documented. ...Gary's platelets rose every day for seven days. From 61,000 to 141,000 strictly from the wheatgrass, nothing else. It's all documented through the lab work. How could someone that ill, with his immune system and his kidneys both shut down, make such a comeback nearly reaching normal blood count? Dr. Smith called it a medical phenomenon. Now, he's taking wheatgrass!

—MRS. GARY (KATHLEEN) GARRETT,
July 1998

Senior Citizen Boosts Body Builders

You wanna hear a story? Call Addison Gold's gym [Bloomingdale, IL]; speak to Mike Niewinski, the manager. Ask him about wheatgrass. ...We can't grow it fast enough for him. ...We sold over 300 trays of grass and 50 juicers. The guys in the gym are going ape over the stuff. They don't need steroids anymore. They feel an energy surge within 15-20 minutes. The bloodstream just sucks that nutrition right in. ...They lift another 20 percent. That's the edge on the competition...they need your sprouts, too. Pea sprouts, broccoli sprouts, sunflower, buckwheat. Your sprout bags are great. It's just amazing stuff. In the past year I've walked in excess of 700 miles across Illinois. I do 2-3 miles per day every day in all weather. I'm telling you it's the wheatgrass. I can't believe my strength. I'll be seventy-two on November 24th.

—LELAND BENDER, Bloomingdale, IL,
written to Steve Meyerowitz[50]

Pretty stunning information, don't you agree? Perhaps the most famous name in wheatgrass history is Ann Wigmore (1909-1994). Author of *The Wheatgrass Book* and co-founder of the Ann Wigmore Foundation (Boston), which has spawned health institutes around the world, Mrs. Wigmore promoted wheatgrass juice as an ideal food to detoxify and replenish the body and also as an alternative cancer treatment. After carrying her message to more than 35 countries, she died unexpectedly from smoke inhalation during a Boston fire. "At the time of her death, she was 84 years young and had more energy than most 20-year-olds!"[51]

Ann Wigmore's story and life work has inspired millions.

To grow wheatgrass you need: 1) wheat seeds, 2) a tray or pot, 3) soil or a growing medium, and 4) water. For best results, most growers use either "hard red winter" or "hard red spring" wheat seeds, but almost any wheat (or barley) seeds will do. Take one to two cups of seeds, place in a jar, and soak overnight (as with most sprouts). After two days of rinsing each morning and evening, when their tiny tails are about one quarter inch long, spread evenly on top of a growing medium (soil, Sure to Grow Pad, even a simple napkin will work) in a tray or pot.

Water moderately, then cover (with either another tray, or even just three to four layers of moist napkins will work). Water directly or mist one or two times a day (directly on the seeds or on the napkins). After two to three days, when the grass blades are coming up nicely, uncover and expose to indoor sunlight. Water your crop daily—again, moist, not drenched. If mold strikes (which happens more easily in warmer temperatures), strike back with a few mists of grapefruit seed extract. In eight to ten days, when the green grass is six or seven inches tall, it's ready for harvest.

The simplest thing to do at this point is to place the cut grass in a blender with water, whiz, strain, and drink. This works. But for best results, *wheatgrass should be juiced*. Some fruit and vegetable juicers can handle wheatgrass too (such as the Omega 8004), but serious wheatgrass drinkers usually invest in a dedicated wheatgrass juicer. Personally, after trying different options, I really like the Hurricane Manual Stainless Steel Wheatgrass Juicer by Handy Pantry. It's sturdy, easy to use, and easy to clean.

Now for a fair warning: Wheatgrass juice is highly-concentrated, chlorophyll-rich, nutrient-loaded *strong stuff*, so start slow. Drink only one or two ounces at a time (at first), and don't be surprised if you experience some "detox symptoms" as your body cleans house. If it's hard to handle the taste, a simple solution is to pour your wheatgrass juice into a glass of fruit juice. This works great for me. No, wheatgrass juice itself isn't as tasty as ice cream, but it won't kill you either. Quite the contrary, it may save your life. You'll get used to it, and the rewards are phenomenal. Free instructional videos, a *How to Grow Sprouts and Wheatgrass* DVD, and complete starter kits are all available at www.wheatgrasskits.com.

If someone you know is critically ill and you don't want to wait to grow your own, there are growers who will overnight to your door either full trays of grass, or flash frozen cubes you just drop into water and drink. In such situations, consider www.dynamicgreens.com (phone: 877-910-0467).

FIGHT BACK WITH GOD'S SPECIAL FORCES

Before the serpent tempted Eve in Eden, God said, "Let the earth bring forth grass" (Gen. 1:11). Whether sprouts, microgreens, or the juice of fresh wheatgrass, all wholesome live foods are God's special forces to fortify our bodies and immune systems with microscopic troops, soldiers, infantry, artillery, and even whole armies to capture, neutralize, defeat, and eliminate deadly bacteria, viruses, pathogens, poisons, toxins, and even mutant, militant, malignant cancer cells. In short, they help our bodies conquer malicious evil agents either created, commissioned, or commanded by the Prince of Disease to undermine and destroy our health.

So fight back with *live food*.

In the battle against deadly diseases, it's a gift of God.

Chapter 10

PURIFICATION IN APOCALYPTIC TIMES

And he said, "Go your way, Daniel, for the words are closed up and sealed till the time of the end. Many shall be purified, made white, and refined, but the wicked shall do wickedly; and none of the wicked shall understand, but the wise shall understand" (Daniel 12:9-10).

Osama bin Laden was mysterious, elusive, cunning, and deadly. Referred to by American media as "a mastermind of evil," he and his highly trained Al Qaeda operatives might strike anytime, anywhere, against anyone, elderly and child alike. Heavily guarded by trusted fellow insurgents, for years he managed to evade US intelligence by hiding deep within dark caves of Afghanistan. Until finally, on May 2, 2011, shortly before 1 A.M. Pakistan time, an elite group of CIA-led Navy Seals of the US Naval Special Warfare Development

Group swept down upon his unsuspecting Pakistani compound. After a brief gunfight, news rang out. "Operation Neptune Spear successful," was the report conveyed to President Obama. "Mission accomplished."

"Osama Bin Laden is dead!"

It was a milestone victory in the war against terror.

Osama Bin Laden may be fitly compared to a mysterious, mutated, metastasizing cancer cell. These microscopic murderers dwelling within our own bodies also strike indiscriminately, against both old and young, even small children. So far, humanity's all-out war against cancer has failed to stop the carnage. Year after year, literally billions of dollars have been raised by the American Cancer Society, the National Cancer Society, the National Breast Cancer Society, and many other societies, foundations, and organizations, to battle cancer and a whole host of other killers, yet millions keep dying. Although significant progress has surely been made, ultimately, so far no wonder drug has been formulated; no magic bullet discovered; and no potion or pill has hit pharmacies, hospitals, or supermarkets that has been proven to consistently and effectively, without toxic side effects, wipe out these devils.

Personally, I believe the all-consuming search for a cure focus is unbalanced. Of course, scientists, doctors, and nutritionists should seek to reverse killer diseases once they start. Not to do so is irresponsible. But it seems to me that the golden key isn't the quest for a cure, but the process of prevention. The truth is, if we can fortify our elite, highly-sophisticated, Navy Seal-type divinely created immune systems by consistently practicing healthy habits, our own bodies can then become cancer killers before these silent invaders gain tactical footholds. But don't forget, we're in the end times. Our enemy is strong, and the battle is on. Notice carefully these words spoken by a holy angel to the prophet Daniel:

> And he said, "Go your way, Daniel, for the words are closed up and sealed till the time of the end. Many shall be purified, made white, and refined, but the wicked shall do wickedly; and none of the wicked shall understand, but the wise shall understand" (Daniel 12:9-10).

This inspired message—communicated directly from heaven—contains life-or-death intelligence information we need to know. In "the time of the end," our greatest survival weapon is to intelligently, conscientiously, and firmly position ourselves among those who "shall be purified." Purified from what? From the evil ways of this fallen world, which include all harmful habits that destroy human health.

Let's review just a bit. Listed below are the Eight Laws of Health. Under each is Lucifer's infernal strategy to kill us and heaven's counterterrorist line of defense.

Nutrition

- *The Devil's Strategy:* To slowly kill us with nutrient-deficient junk food.

- *God's Plan of Defense:* More raw plant foods, fresh juices, live foods.

Exercise

- *The Devil's Strategy:* Make us immobile, lazy couch potatoes.

- *God's Plan of Defense:* Keep all muscles moving. Use it or lose it.

Water

- *The Devil's Strategy:* Alcohol, coffee, and sugar-loaded sodas.

- *God's Plan of Defense:* Drink more pure, clean, life-giving water.

Sunlight

- *The Devil's Strategy:* Stay indoors, mostly in artificial light; avoid the sun.

- *God's Plan of Defense:* Lots of sunlight (without overdoing it) resulting in abundant vitamin D production.

Temperance

- *The Devil's Strategy:* If it tastes good, swallow it. Taste buds rule.

- *God's Plan of Defense:* In His strength, say no to all health-destroying substances. "Moderation in what is good, abstain from what is harmful."

Fresh Air

- *The Devil's Strategy:* Pollute lungs and bloodstreams with marijuana, tobacco, and smog. Keep all windows closed; breathe stale air, always.

- *God's Plan of Defense:* Open windows often. Breathe deep, fresh air.

Rest

- *The Devil's Strategy:* Overwork. Stay up late. Never take a vacation.

- *God's Plan of Defense:* Get a good night's sleep. Rest body and brain.

Trust God

- *The Devil's Strategy:* False science. Evolution from apes. Atheism.

- *God's Plan of Defense:* Realize that a Master Designer formed our bodies. Our Creator loves us. Repent. Trust. Obey. His will is for our best good. Be pure. Maintain a clean conscience. Be thankful.

Two days after the Twin Towers in New York City imploded into oblivion on September 11, 2001, President George W. Bush declared, "The most important thing is for us to find Osama bin Laden." "It is our number-one priority," he added, "and we will not rest until we find him."[52]

Sometimes truth is like the nose on our face. It's right in front of us, yet we can't see it. It's the same with the Eight Laws of Health. They aren't hard to understand, and from a health standpoint they are the number-one issue of our generation. To win this war, discovering and following them should be our top priority. God realizes this; thus His end-time strategy involves teaching and separating His people from all sinful and unhealthy habits and bringing them into harmony with immutable divine laws, both natural and moral.

The Eight Laws are God's health laws. The Ten Commandments are God's moral laws. Both laws overlap. Both are sacred. Health Law number eight, Trusting God, places our Maker where He should be—center stage in our lives—which is the same as keeping the first commandment that states, "You shall have no other gods before Me" (Exod. 20:3). Unhealthy habits can easily become idols, which violates commandment two forbidding idolatry (see Exod. 20:4-6). The sixth commandment, "You shall not murder" (Exod. 20:13), also applies to slow self-murder by harmful habits. Thus we can see clearly that God's moral and health laws fit together like a lock and a key. So what is His program today? The book of Daniel pinpoints the answer. His plan is *to purify a people in "the time of the end."*

Echoing perfectly the Old Testament prophecy of Daniel 12:9-10, the apostle Paul in the New Testament summarized the glorious goals of grace:

> *For the grace of God that brings salvation has appeared to all men, teaching us that, denying ungodliness and worldly lusts, we should live soberly, righteously, and godly in the present age, looking for the blessed hope and glorious appearing of our great God and Savior Jesus Christ, who gave Himself for us, that He might redeem us from every lawless deed and purify for Himself His own special people, zealous for good works* (Titus 2:11-14).

There it is. First, Paul says that "the grace of God" is now available to "all men." Thank the Lord. We've all sinned and need His forgiveness. Next, Paul reveals that true grace teaches us to deny (which means saying "No!") all "ungodliness" and "worldly lusts," which include all unnatural passions and desires, in this "present age" of slick advertising, alluring temptation, addictive cravings, sexual perversity, nutrient-deficient junk foods, and peer pressure. Honestly, we can't overcome these evils in our own strength, which is why Jesus Christ has become our "Savior." He "gave Himself for us." How marvelous! He gave everything—even His own life—when He willingly sacrificed Himself on a cruel cross to atone for our sins.

Why did He do it? What was His goal? To leave us in sin, controlled by lust and the devil? No! Look closely: "that He might redeem us from every lawless deed and purify for Himself His own special people, zealous for good works." Thus God's ultimate agenda is to "purify for Himself" a group of helpless sinners, rescuing them "from every lawless deed," and thus bringing them into harmony with His divine laws, both natural and moral. This elite group will be fully prepared for the "glorious appearing"—the Second Coming of Jesus Christ.

"Many will be purified," predicted the angel. *Many* means some, but not all. Sadly, the majority would rather lazily wallow in their lusts. They refuse to fight. But those who are willing to take a stand, battle their own bodies, and even their own taste buds will not only be healthier, happier, and save money in medical bills, but they will significantly decrease their chances of dropping dead early in the Great War. Above all, they will be better able to serve King Jesus, who sacrificed

His precious life for our sins. This is the highest motivation to be healthy and holy. Then we can fulfill the Scripture which states, "For you were bought at a price; therefore *glorify God* in your body and in your spirit, which are God's" (1 Cor. 6:20).

During earthly wars, such as in Afghanistan, many brave soldiers have had their bodies blasted by explosions from hidden bombs. In some cases, amputating an arm or leg is the only option for survival. The same principle applies in the war against our health. *But I love this bad habit,* some may be thinking. Yes, you may enjoy it or even think you need it, but if it has become a deadly devilish weapon to destroy your health, the wiser voice of your conscience should be summoning you to change course. "Time to amputate." urges the Great Physician. "Many shall be purified," penned His prophet. So take the knife. Make the sacrifice. Slice off the enemy. Your body will reward you if you do.

Let me again clarify, in this fallen world being stricken with some form of sickness is often unavoidable due to human ignorance, environmental factors, or genetics. Ultimately, death itself is inevitable, primarily because Adam and Eve listened to Lucifer and committed sin in Paradise. So please, don't get a wrong impression from this book that whenever a person gets sick it's their own fault and they are to blame. Sometimes it is. Sometimes it isn't. Life is complex. There are some things we have no control over. Nevertheless, the message of *End Times Health War* is that there is much we *can* do to decisively win many battles, survive, and stay alive—at least for a while.

According to the Holy Bible, our greatest hope is not the National Institutes of Health, the Institute of Medicine, well-funded research scientists, that medical professionals will finally discover a cure for cancer, or even that we will remain disease-free for the next 50 to 100 years. Instead, it's Jesus Christ's return. "Behold, He is coming with clouds," predicts the Book of God, "and every eye will see Him" (Rev. 1:7). "Behold, I am coming quickly! Blessed is he who keeps the words of the prophecy of this book" (Rev. 22:7).

> *I am the Alpha and the Omega, the Beginning and the End, the First and the Last. Blessed are those who do His commandments, that they may have the right to the tree of life, and may enter through the gates into the city [the New Jerusalem]. ...The grace of our Lord Jesus Christ be with you all. Amen* (Revelation 22:13-14,21).

The end times have arrived. Heaven's clock is ticking. These are the last days. The Day of the Lord is near. "The time is at hand" (Rev. 22:10). As we strive to stay alive in this perilous apocalyptic age and as we wait for His return, no matter what happens we can still comfort ourselves with the good news that:

1. When sickness does strike, our loving Creator is ready, willing, and able to "[comfort] us in all our tribulation, that we may be able to comfort those who are in any trouble" (2 Cor. 1:4). He is the "Father of mercies and God of all comfort" (2 Cor. 1:3).

2. When Jesus Christ returns "in the glory of His Father with His angels" (Matt. 16:27), He will "transform our lowly body that it may be

conformed to His glorious body" (Phil. 3:21). Paul described it this way: "In a moment, in the twinkling of an eye, at the last trumpet. For the trumpet will sound, and the dead will be raised incorruptible, and we shall be changed. For this corruptible must put on incorruption, and this mortal must put on immortality" (1 Cor. 15:52-53). From corruption to immortality. How sweet the thought. No more sore backs, aching bones, fading eyesight, gray hair, wrinkled skin, or wheelchairs. Alleluia!

3. After "the day of the Lord" when God finally detoxifies His polluted planet from every trace of evil, when "the heavens will pass away with a great noise, and the elements will melt with fervent heat," His saints will joyfully witness the long-awaited literal fulfillment of "His promise" to create "new heavens and a new earth in which righteousness dwells" (2 Pet. 3:10,13). It will be Eden restored!

4. All suffering will then cease forever, as it is written, "'And God will wipe away every tear from their eyes; there shall be no more death, nor sorrow, nor crying. There shall be no more pain, for the former things have passed away.' Then He who sat on the throne said, 'Behold, I make all things new.' And He said to me, 'Write, for these words are true and faithful'" (Rev. 21:4-5). No more ambulance sirens, paramedics, hospitals,

hospice organizations, graveside services, or tear-filled funerals. Again, alleluia!

5. Lucifer will be gone. "The devil, who deceived them [the lost], was cast into the lake of fire and brimstone" (Rev. 20:10). Jesus Himself will "destroy him who had the power of death, that is, the devil" (Heb. 2:14). "I destroyed you," God predicted in Old Testament times, "O covering cherub...I turned you to ashes...you have become a horror, and shall be no more forever" (Ezek. 28:16,18-19). No more temptations. No demons. No more devil.

6. The Great War will be over. "The last enemy that will be destroyed is death" (1 Cor. 15:26). When the smoke clears and the dust settles, "every creature which is in heaven and on the earth and under the earth and such as are in the sea, and all that are in them, I heard saying: 'Blessing and honor and glory and power be to Him who sits on the throne, and to the Lamb, forever and ever!'" (Rev. 5:13).

7. Living in the light of the eternal Presence of God, the Lord's redeemed people will be holy, happy, and healthy forever. "And there shall be no more curse, but the throne of God and of the Lamb shall be in it [inside the New Jerusalem], and His servants shall serve Him. They shall see His face, and His name shall be on their foreheads.

...They need no lamp nor light of the sun, for the Lord God gives them light. And they shall reign forever and ever" (Rev. 22:3-5). "And He who sits on the throne will dwell among them. They shall neither hunger anymore nor thirst anymore; the sun shall not strike them, nor any heat; for the Lamb who is in the midst of the throne will shepherd them and lead them to living fountains of water. And God will wipe away every tear from their eyes" (Rev. 7:15-17).

On March 3, 2013, our son Seth woke up early and rushed into our living room in Idaho where I sat warming myself by a newly stoked fire. "Daddy," he blurted out excitedly, "I had a dream last night!"

"What did you dream?" I replied curiously.

"In my dream I was taken up to the holy city. I saw the streets of gold. Then I saw Jesus sitting on His throne. Daddy, Jesus was so bright, I had to squint to look at Him!" *That's amazing,* I thought to myself. He then drew a picture of his dream on a piece of paper and signed it, "Seth. 3-3-13." Put it on Facebook," he then suggested with a boyish grin, which I did.

FYI, my Facebook group knows about Seth's battle with seizures. Many have prayed for him too. In fact, people around the world have prayed for our son, and I believe that their prayers are a key part of his progress in our family's struggle for his health.

Dear reader, God is real. Heaven is real too. "These words are true and faithful" (Rev. 21:5), promises our King from His throne. In the midst of your own personal health battles, take heart. Though the warfare seems long and fierce and temptation or illness strong, don't be afraid. God loves you. He is mighty. He will help you, one step at a time. If you fall down, get up. If you yield to temptation, don't sink into self-pity. Trust Jesus and try again. In the midst of discouragement, look beyond this short life's aches and pains to a vast eternity beyond. Even if we die and rest for a while in a grave, the Risen One promises those who believe in Him, "I will raise him up at the last day" (John 6:44). "I am the resurrection and the life" (John 11:25). Our merciful Savior has not only conquered Satan, sin, and sickness, but Death itself. Jesus Himself is the Almighty Victor in the Great War.

On His new earth, where "a pure river of water of life, clear as crystal" flows constantly "from the throne of God and of the Lamb" (see Rev. 22:1), there "the inhabitant will not say, 'I am sick'; [and] the people who dwell [there] will be forgiven their iniquity" (Isa. 33:24).

I hope to see you there.

Appendix A

VITAMIN B12: DON'T LEAVE HOME WITHOUT IT

As *End Times Health War* was preparing to go to press, I received this stirring testimony from one of my endorsers, Dr. Timothy Arnott, MD, about the critical importance of Vitamin B12, and decided it was worth adding in an Appendix to this book. From a health standpoint, vitamin B12 and vitamin D parallel each other in that, although both are labeled as "vitamins," they do not naturally occur in plant food, but are essential. As we know, vitamin D is produced by the body from sunlight, whereas B12 is primarily produced by lowly bacteria in the mouth and colon. Although it has myriads of critical functions, B12 is particularly essential *for the health of the brain*—God's highest creation on earth. Thus the most complex organ (the brain) is dependent on some of the lowliest organisms (bacteria), which contains a grand lesson in itself. In these end times—for some insidious reason that the devil is no doubt involved with—getting enough B12 has also become a serious and life-threatening global problem, even for those who adopt an ideal diet. Thus B12 too is within the war zone. Based on this, here is Dr. Timothy Arnott's timely message:

As a physician in private practice for 20 years, I have discovered a consistent pattern among my American patients. Namely, total and LDL cholesterol are always high and vitamin D and vitamin B12 are almost always low. I also have a number of Seventh-day Adventists as patients. They are a group featured in a National Geographic article, "The Secrets of Long Life ," by Dan Buettner[1] as one of three groups world-wide that excel in longevity. Approximately 36% of this group are vegetarian.[2] Included in this group are many vegan Adventists too,[3] perhaps the largest sub-group of vegans in this country. A high percentage of my Seventh-day Adventist patients are vegan or near-vegan. Among these patients, I have noticed another pattern. They have ideal total cholesterol and LDL cholesterol levels.[4]

However, to my surprise, their vitamin D and vita-min B12 levels are even lower than my patients who eat animal products. This finding is not unique to my medical practice.[5,6] Over 200 scientific articles have documented vegans to have the lowest vitamin B12 levels in the world,[7] and they also have the highest homocysteine levels among the general population.[8,9] Why is this important? First, it should be noted that low vitamin B12 status does not undo all the bene-fits of a vegan or vegetarian diet. This is underscored by the fact that vegetarian and vegan Adventists still have the greatest longevity of any other group reported in the medical literature.[10] However, this vegetarian and vegan longevity advantage could be even greater if these individuals took a simple vitamin B12 supplement daily, for the rest of their lives.

The possible medical consequences of low vitamin B12 blood levels (high homocysteine) are not to be ignored. Namely, weakened immune system,[11] memory loss,[12] dementia,[13] anemia,[14] neuropathy,[15] unsteady gait,[16] loss of pregnancy,[17] seizures,[18] cardiovascular disease,[19] abdominal aortic aneurysm,[20] and, when coupled with low vitamin D levels, cancer.[21] Therefore, we all do ourselves a great service of avoiding all these potential catastrophic adverse health outcomes by daily chewing a sublingual vitamin B12 [methylcobalamin] supplement, 1000-2000mcg. I also recommend that everyone obtain a vitamin B12 blood test before taking vitamin B12. If you do, you will likely be told your level is in the "normal" range, and your physician may tell you your B12 level is fine. They may be wrong.[22] They are probably practicing medicine based on currently established reference ranges, which are based on population samples, not based on optimal levels for health.[23] My advice is to make sure your vitamin B12 level is at the top of the reference range, not near the bottom, namely, at 1100 pg/ml. If you want the lowest homocysteine level in the population, bring your B12 level up even as high as 1400 pg/ml, and keep your homocysteine level below 7.2 umol/L.[24] With adequate B12 supplementation, and God's help, you may be able to reach this goal of having your B12 level at 1400 pg/ml.[25]

Vitamin B12 is especially important for pregnant mothers,[26] nursing moms, and growing children.[27] You cannot divide a cell without vitamin B12. In other words, you cannot sustain a pregnancy without adequate B12. You also need B12 to create the myelin sheath insulation around your nerves.[28] Thus I urge you, please, to take vitamin B12 seriously. It will ensure that if you do adapt a plant-based diet (due to its fabulous health benefits) you will also avoid any adverse outcomes closely tied to B12 deficiency.

TIMOTHY JON ARNOTT, MD
Board-certified, Family Medicine
Founding Member, American College of Lifestyle Medicine

For more information on the vital importance of vitamin B12, see the book, *Could It Be B12?: An Epidemic of Misdiagnosis,* by Sally M. Pacholok, R.N., B.S.N., and Jeffrey J. Stuart, D.O.

Appendix A References

1. Dan Buettner, "The Secrets of a Long Life," *National Geographic Magazine,* November 2005.

2. M. J. Orlich, "Vegetarian Dietary Patterns and Mortality in Adventist Health Study 2," JAMA Internal Medicine 173, no. 13 (2013):1230-1238.

3. Ibid.

4. C. B. Esselstyn, "Changing the Treatment Paradigm for Coronary Artery Disease," American Journal of Cardiology 82, no. 10B (1998):2T-4T.

5. C. J. Hung, "Plasma Homocysteine Levels in Taiwanese Vegetarians are Higher than those of Omnivores," Journal of Nutrition 132, no. 2 (2002):152-8.

6. L. T. Ho Pham, "Vegetarianism, Bone Loss, Fracture and Vitamin D: A Longitudinal Study in Asian Vegans and Non-vegans," European Journal of Clinical Nutrition 66, no. 1 (2012):75-82.

7. http://www.ncbi.nlm.nih.gov/pubmed/?term=vegan+AND+b12

8. http://www.ncbi.nlm.nih.gov/pubmed/?term=vegan+AND+homocysteine

9. C. J. Hung, "Plasma Homocysteine Levels,":152-8.

10. G. Frazer, "Ten Years of Life – Is it a Matter of Choice?" Archives of Internal Medicine 161 (2001):1645-1652.

11. F. T. Fata, "Impaired Antibody Responses to Pneumococcal Polysaccharide in Elderly Patients with Low Serum Vitamin B12 Levels," Annals of Internal Medicine 124, no. 3 (1996):299-304.

12. N. Iqtidar, "Misdiagnosed Vitamin B12 Deficiency a Challenge to be Confronted by Use of Modern Screening Markers," Journal of the Pakistan Medical Association 62, no. 11 (2012):1223-9.

13. Ibid.

14. M. J. Oberley, "Laboratory Testing for Cobalmin Deficiency in Megaloblastic Anemia," American Journal of Hematology 88, no. 6 (2013):522-6.

15. N. Kumar, "Neurologic Aspects of Cobalamin (B12) Deficiency," Handbook of Clinical Neurology 120 (2014):915-26.

16. J. R. Crawford, D. Say, "Vitamin B12 Deficiency Presenting as Acute Ataxia," BMJ Case Reports (March 26, 2013).

17. HU. Hubner, "Low Serum Vitamin B12 is Associated with Recurrent Pregnancy Loss in Syrian Women," Clinical Chemistry and Laboratory Medicine 46, no. 9 (2008):1265-9.

18. M. Dogan, S. Ariyuca, E. Peker, S. Akbayram, S. Z. Dogan, O. Ozdemir, Y. Cesur, "Psychotic Disorder, Hypertension and Seizures Associated with Vitamin B12 Deficiency: A Case Report," Human & Experimental Toxicology 31, no. 4 (2012):410-3.

19. S. C. Tyagi, "Homocyst(e)ine and Heart Disease: Pathophysiology of Extracellular Matrix," Clinical and Experimental Hypertension 21, no. 3 (1999):181-98.

20. Y. Y. Wong, J. Golledge, L. Flicker, K. A. McCaul, G. J. Hankey, F. M. van Bockxmeer, B. B. Yeap, P. E. Norman, "Plasma Total Homocysteine is Associated with Abdominal Aortic Aneurysm and Aortic Diameter in Older men," Journal of Vascular Surgery 58, no. 2 (2013):364-70.

21. D. Divisi, S. Di Tommaso, S. Salvemini, M. Garramone, R. Crisci, "Diet and Cancer," Acta Biomedica 77, no. 2 (2006):118-23.

22. N. Iqtidar, "Misdiagnosed Vitamin B12 Deficiency," 1223-9

23. Ibid.

24. J. Tayama, Hypertension Research 29, no. 6 (2006):403-9.

25. N. J. Mann, "The Effect of Diet on Plasma Homocysteine Concentrations in Healthy Male Subjects," European Journal of Clinical Nutrition 53, no. 11 (1999):895-9.

26. A. M. Molloy, "Effects of Folate and Vitamin B12 Deficiencies During Preganancy on Fetal, Infant, and Child Development," Food and Nutrition Bulletin 29 (2008):S101-11.

27. D. Aleksic, D. Djokic, I. Golubicic, V. Jakovljevic, D. Djuric, "The Importance of the Blood Levels of Homocysteine, Folic Acid and Vitamin B12 in Children with Malignant Diseases, "Journal of BUON 18, no 4 (2013):1019-25.

28. A. J. Miller, Journal of the Neurological Sciences 233, no. 12 (2005):93-7.

RECOMMENDED READING

Health Smart: A Rational, No-Nonsense Practical Approach to Health, by Walter C. Thompson, M.D.

Dr. Arnott's 24 Realistic Ways to Improve Your Health, by Tim Arnott, M.D.

Proof Positive: How to Reliably Combat Disease and Achieve Optimal Health through Nutrition and Lifestyle, by Neil Nedley, M.D.

The China Study: Startling Implications for Diet, Weight Loss and Long Term Health, by T. Colin Campbell, Ph.D., and Thomas M. Campbell II.

Fasting and Eating for Health: A Medical Doctor's Program for Conquering Disease, by Joel Fuhrman, M.D.

Detoxify or Die, by Sherry A. Rogers, M.D.

Suicide by Sugar: A Startling Look at Our #1 National Addiction, by Nancy Appleton, Ph.D

The Ministry of Healing, by Ellen G. White

The Magnesium Miracle, by Carolyn Dean, M.D., N.D.

Iodine: Why You Need It, Why You Can't Live Without It, by David Brownstein, M.D.

The Healing Power of Chlorophyll from Plant Life, by Bernard Jensen, D.C., Ph.D., Nutritionist

Sprout Garden: Indoor Growers Guide to Gourmet Sprouts, by Mark M. Braunstein

Wheatgrass, Sprouts, Microgreens, and the Living Food Diet, by Living Whole Foods, Inc.

The Wheatgrass Book: How to Grow and Use Wheatgrass to Maximize Your Health and Vitality, by Ann Wigmore

The Healing Crisis, by Bruce Fife

The Green Pharmacy Guide to Healing Foods: Proven Natural Remedies to Treat and Prevent More than 80 Common Health Concerns, by James A. Duke, PhD

Charcoal Remedies.com: The Complete Handbook of Medicinal Charcoal and Its Applications, by John Dinsley

The Narrow Road of Natural Healing, by Linda Clark

Add Life, a gluten-free vegetarian cookbook and nutrition guide, by Sheri Yohe

Notes

Introduction

1. CBC News, "World Cancer Deaths to Double by 2030: UN," CBC News Technology & Science, June 02, 2010, http://www.cbc.ca/news/technology/world-cancer-deaths-to-double-by-2030-un-1.938651.

2. Zosia Chustecka, "Cancer Strikes 1 in 2 Men and 1 in 3 Women," Medscape Multispeciality, February 9, 2007, http://www.medscape.com/viewarticle/551998.

Chapter 4:
End Times Report: Planet Earth Is Toxic

3. Duff Wilson, "Fear in the Fields: How Hazardous Waste Becomes Fertilizer," *The Seattle Times*, July 3-4, 1997, http://seattletimes.com/news/special/fear_fields.html.

4. Neil K. Kaneshiro, "Death Among Children and Adolescents," Medline, http://nim.nih.gov/medlineplus/ency/article/001915.htm.

5. "Fourth National Report on Human Exposure to Environmental Chemicals, 2009," Centers for Disease Control and Prevention, http://www.cdc.gov/exposurereport/pdf/FourthReport_ExecutiveSummary.pdf (accessed February 20, 2014).

6. "Mercury: Health Effects," Environmental Protection Agency, http://www.epa.gov/mercury/effects.htm.

7. "Introduction to Indoor Air: Lead," Environmental Protection Agency, http://www.epa.gov/iaq/lead.htm.

8. "Arsenic in Drinking Water," Environmental Protection Agency, http://www.epa.gov/lawsregs/rulesregs/sdwa/arsenic/index.cfm.

9. "Radiation Protection: Uranium,"

Environmental Protection Agency, http://www.epa.gov/rpdweb00/radionuclides/uranium.html.

10. "Toxic Substances Portal: Cadmium," Agency for Toxic Substances & Disease Registry, http://www.astsdr.cdc.gov/substances/toxsubstance.asp?toxid+15.

11. http://www.huffingtonpost.com/bill-chameides/the-chemical-marketplace_b_1317149.html.

12. Bryan Walsh, "The Plight of the Honeybee," *Time*, August 19, 2013, 26.

13. Ibid., 27.

14. Ibid.

CHAPTER 5: PUT ON THE WHOLE ARMOR OF GOD

15. Joe White and Nicholas Comninellis, *Darwin's Demise* (Green Forest, AR: Master Books, 2001), 29-30.

CHAPTER 6: EIGHT WEAPONS FOR WINNING THE WAR

16. Deborah Kotz, "11 Healthy Habits that Will Help You Live to 100," U. S. News & World Report, http://health.usnews.com/health-news/family/living-well/articles/2009/02/20/10-health-habits-that-will-help-you-live-to-100?page+2.

17. Rudy Davis, ND, "Ancient Elixir Rediscovered," YouTube, August 7, 2013, http://www.youtube.com/watch?v =5Hb_4DXMMsU.

18. Michael F. Holick, *The Vitamin D Solution* (New York, NY: Hudson Street Press, 2010), 244.

19. "What Is Vitamin D?" Vitamin D Council, http://www .vitamindcouncil.org/about-vitamin-d/what-is-vitamin-d/. (accessed February 23, 2014).

20. Holick, *The Vitamin D Solution,* xviii.

21. Soram Khalsa, *The Vitamin D Revolution* (Carlsbad, CA: Hay House, 2009), 66.

22. Mark Stibich, "Top 10 Health Benefits of a Good Night's Sleep," About.com Healthy Aging, May 8, 2009, http:// longevity.about.com/od/lifelongenergy/tp/healthy_sleep .htm.

23. Maureen Mackey, "Sleepless in America: A \$32.4 Billion Business," The Fiscal Times, July 23, 2012, http://www.thefiscaltimes.com/Articles/2012/07/23/ Sleepless-in-America-A-32-4-Billion-Business.

24. Ellen G. White, *Counsels on Health* (Mountain View, CA: Pacific Press Pub. Association, 1951), 628.

CHAPTER 7: SPECIAL FORCES: FRESH, RAW JUICES

25. "It's Easy to Add Fruits and Vegetables to Your Diet," American Cancer Society, October 16, 2013, http:// www.cancer.org/healthy/eathealthygetactive/eathealthy/ add-fruits-and-veggies-to-your-diet.

26. "Synopsis," Fat, Sick & Nearly Died, http://www .fatsickand nearlydead.com/about.html.

27. "About NutritionFacts.org," NutritionFacts.org, http:// nutritionfacts.org/about/. (accessed February 25, 2014).

28. Dr. Michael Greger, Smoking Versus Kale Juice," Nutritionfacts.org, March 8, 2012, http://nutritionfacts .org/video/smoking-versus-kale-juice/.

29. A. Vanhatalo et al., "Acute and Chronic Effects of Dietary Nitrate Supplementation on Blood Pressure and the Physiological Responses to Moderate-intensity and Incremental Exercise," *AJP: Regulatory, Integrative and Comparative Physiology* 299, no. 4 (August 30, 2010): abstract, doi:10.1152/ajpregu.00206.2010.

30. Brenda Davis, Vesanto Melina, and Rynn Berry, *Becoming Raw* (Summertown, TN: Book Pub., 2010), 52.

31. Steven Prussack and Bo Rinaldi, *The Complete Idiot's Guide to Juice Fasting (New York, NY: Alpha Books, 2012), 202.*

32. Ibid., 201.

33. Richard Schulze, *There Are No Incurable Diseases* (Santa Monica, CA: Natural Healing Publications, 1999), 25.

34. Prussack and Rinaldi, *The Complete Idiot's Guide to Juice Fasting*, 196.

35. Ravi, "The Best Product," Amazon.com, August 21, 2012, http://www.amazon.com/review/R1E5UIQ5C9XK9Y/ ref%3Dcm_cr_rdp_perm?ie=UTF8&ASIN =B001RLYOEE&linkCode=&nodeID=&tag=.

36. Albert J. Valentino, "Why It's the Best Value Juicer on the Market," Amazon.com, June 17, 2012, http:// www.amazon.com/review/RHX1KFWM3SC50/ ref=cm_cr_rdp_perm?ie=UTF8&ASIN =B001RLYOEE&linkCode=&nodeID=&tag=.

37. Aaron, "Review of Omega J8004," Amazon.com, accessed February 26, 2014, http://www.amazon.com/ review/R1EFBP4X8GYD33ref=cm_cr_pr_cmtie =UTF8&ASIN=B001RLYOEE&linkCode =&nodeID=&tag=#wasThisHelpful.

38. Mr. Perfectionist, "Great Buy. Juicing Changed My Life," Amazon.com, January 31, 2012, http://www.amazon. com/review/R136TP2KMVRQ20/ref=cm_cr_rdp_perm ?ie=UTF8&ASIN =B001RLYOEE&linkCode=&nodeID =&tag=.

CHAPTER 8: STRUGGLES, DISCOVERIES, VICTORIES

39. White, *Counsels on Health*, 324.

CHAPTER 9: MORE SPECIAL FORCES: SPROUT POWER

40. Crystal Gammon, "Weed Killer Kills Human Cells. Study Intensifies Debate over 'inert' Ingredients," Environmental Health News, June 22, 2009, http://www. environmentalhealthnews.org/ehs/news/roundup -weed-killer-is-toxic-to-human-cells.-study-intensifies -debate-over-inert-ingredients.

41. Ibid.

42. "The EPA and Food Security," EPA, http://www.epa.gov/ pesticides/factsheets/securty.htm. (accessed May 26, 2012)

43. "Cancer Trends Progress Report: Pesticides," National Cancer Institute, June 20, 2012, http:// www.progressreport.cancer.gov/doc_detail.asp ?pid=1&did=2007&chid=71&coid=713&mid.

44. LaSalle D. Leffall, Jr., Margaret L. Kripke, "Reducing Environmental Cancer Risk: What We Can Do Now, 2008-2009 Annual Report," National Cancer Institute, http://deainfo.nci.nih.gov/advisory/pcp/annualReports/pcp08-09rpt/PCP_Report_08-09_508.pdf.

45. Steve Meyerowitz, *Sprouts, the Miracle Food: The Complete Guide to Sprouting* (Great Barrington, MA: Sproutman Publications, 1999), 7-8.

46. Ibid., 93.

47. Davis, *Becoming Raw,* 142.

48. Nita Mukherjee, "Composition and Health Benefits of Sprouts," Suites, August 9, 2009, https://suite101.com/a/composition-and-health-benefits-of-sprouts-a137716.

49. Jennifer Warner, "Tiny Microgreens Packed with Nutrients," WebMD, August 31, 2012, http://www.webmd.com/diet/news/20120831/tiny-microgreens-packed-nutrients.

50. Meyerowitz, Steve, *Wheatgrass: Nature's Finest Medicine*, 7th ed. (Great Barrington, MA: Sproutman Publications, 2006), 105-136.

51. "About the Institute: Dr. Ann Wigmore," Ann Wigmore Natural Health Institute, http://annwigmore.org/about.html (accessed February 28, 2014).

CHAPTER 10: PURIFICATION IN APOCALYPTIC TIMES

52. "Osama Bin Laden: Timeline," Atlanta Journal-Constitution, May 3, 2011, http://www.ajc.com/news/news/national/osama-bin-laden-timeline-1/nQs9R/.

ABOUT STEVE WOHLBERG

Steve Wohlberg is the speaker/director of White Horse Media (Priest River, Idaho) and the host of *His Voice Today* radio and television broadcasts. He is the author of 30-plus books, has been a guest on over 500 radio shows, has been featured in three History Channel documentaries (*Secrets of the Seven Seals; Strange Rituals: Apocalypse; Armageddon Battle Plan*) one National Geographic International documentary (*Animal Apocalypse*), and has spoken by special invitation inside the Pentagon and US Senate. He currently lives in Priest River, Idaho with his lovely wife, Kristin, and their two children, Seth Michael and Abigail Rose. His ministry website is www.whitehorsemedia.com.